THE CHEAT SYSTEM DIET

THE
CHEAT
SYSTEM DIET

Eat the Foods You Crave
and Lose Weight Even Faster

JACKIE WICKS

Founder of PEERtrainer

St. Martin's Press ❧ New York

This book contains information and recommendations based on scientific research. However, it is not intended to provide medical advice, and it should not replace the guidance of a qualified physician or other healthcare provider. Decisions about your health should be made by you and your healthcare provider based on the specific circumstances of your health, risk factors, family history, and other considerations. See your healthcare provider before making major dietary changes or embarking on an exercise program, especially if you have existing health problems, medical conditions, or chronic diseases.

www.stmartins.com

Designed by Patrice Sheridon

Photo on page 37, courtesy of Joel Fuhrman, M.D., author of *Eat to Live Cookbook*
Photos on pages 71–79, courtesy of Egoscue Inc.
Photos on pages 317–320, courtesy of Z-Health Performance Solutions, LLC

LIBRARY OF CONGRESS CATALOGING-IN-PUBLICATION DATA

Wicks, Jackie.
   The cheat system diet : eat the foods you crave and lose weight even faster / Jackie Wicks, founder of PEERtrainer.
      pages cm
   ISBN 978-1-250-04469-3 (hardcover)
   ISBN 978-1-4668-4316-5 (e-book)
   1. Weight loss.   2. Exercise.   3. Nutrition.   4. Food preferences.   5. Self-care, Health.   I. Title.
   RM222.2.W4524 2014
   613.2'5—dc23

                                                                2014007509

St. Martin's Press books may be purchased for educational, business, or promotional use. For information on bulk purchases, please contact Macmillan Corporate and Premium Sales Department at 1-800-221-7945, extension 5442, or write specialmarkets@macmillan.com.

First Edition: May 2014

10   9   8   7   6   5   4   3   2   1

Contents

Introduction: Why You Can't Lose Weight Now

Welcome. I'm so excited to share the Cheat System with you because I know you'll find relief in these pages. There is a lot of pain and frustration out there for people who are struggling with their weight; I hear it every day. Dieting has become so confusing, so regimented, so contradictory that people become defeated within days of trying something new or even before they start. As the founder of the Web site PEERtrainer.com, I get e-mails and hear from readers that say, "I've already cheated this morning. My day is shot. What's the point?"

I used to think the same thing. I would get up, be late, need "energy" for a meeting, and get a bacon-egg-and-cheese sandwich and a large latte. In that moment, I would think, "Ugh, I cheated again." And I would beat myself up. I wanted to lose weight so badly. I was determined to get back into my pre-pregnancy clothes—so why was I cheating again?

It took me a long time to realize and understand that the most important thing to remember about weight loss is that there should always be some room for mistakes and slip-ups. Beating myself up over a mistake at breakfast didn't get me anywhere but possibly led to another bad choice at lunch or gave me an excuse to skip the gym and hang out on the sofa.

So I started to think, What could work? What could I actually do? What plan would actually work? What diet plan could I do where I could lose weight and still go out to dinner and eat without feeling guilty?

What would people like me actually do, not just for one week, not just for two weeks, not just for three weeks? What would people like me actually do, day in and day out, without getting frustrated or discouraged the moment they slipped up by having cheese and crackers?

When people cheat on their diets, they quit. But they still desperately want a plan that works—one that helps them lose weight and get healthy. Any plan that works in real life has to keep people from quitting. A plan that works in real life has to allow for slip-ups and Cheats and making mistakes—and birthday parties!

I've spent the last eight years obsessed with one question: What diet will people actually follow through with? People want to stick to a program and achieve their weight and health goals, and I wanted to find the diet that will help them actually do it. I've been *obsessed* with finding the combination of habits and practices that will help people stick to what they want to do: lose weight, be healthy, and feel good.

If most popular diet and fitness regimens actually worked, we wouldn't be continually frustrated and have such an impossible time losing weight. The information many of these plans provide isn't bad (although in some cases it is; and sometimes it's egregious—more on that later). The problem is that most of these programs are easy when you're psyched or motivated. But what about when you're not? When you're overwhelmed or stressed? When your boss hands you something at 5 p.m., when your husband has to work late *again*, when you get in a fight with your sister, or your babysitter cancels? Then the rules become impossible. And that's when we resort to our old habits that won't help us lose weight, but ultimately are easy—and we need easy when the tsunami of the world overwhelms us.

Whatever the plan is—even if it has the best information available—if you don't put it into action it might as well just be a movie. Afterward you think, "Wow, that looked really great. Wish I could do that/go there/be that person." That's why I'm obsessed with follow-through—the only plan that will change your life and body is the one you'll actually do.

The information out there about weight loss is so complicated that asking you to figure out what will work is like asking you to lift a hundred-pound weight. Maybe one day you'll be ready, but if I asked you to lift that weight right now, I'd be overwhelming your body. I've designed this book to be like a five-pound starter weight: something you can handle.

What you'll learn in this book is the opposite of what most people think "works" for weight loss. For example, you'll learn that **portion control can't work alone**—because most of the time, people can't follow through on a portion control plan no matter how well intentioned.

If people feel hungry, they'll "cheat" and feel so guilty, they quit. The truth, as you'll learn in the next chapter, is that you only have to monitor how much you eat of *some* foods, not everything you eat. **You can eat as much as you want of many foods and still lose weight!** I'll also prove that **the "no pain, no gain" mantra about exercise is completely wrong.** Working out that way can actually hold you *back* from becoming fitter, faster, and stronger because it pushes our body past the limit where we burn fat and activates stress hormones that can actually add weight on.

So who am I and why should you take advice from me? In 2004, I was a new mom of a baby boy, and I realized I had only lost twenty pounds from the peak of my pregnancy weight, which was 185 pounds. (I'm five feet five inches.) After months of being at 165, I knew that I wasn't going to be one of the lucky ones for whom breastfeeding took off the weight. I was so frustrated—I knew what I had to do, but I just wasn't doing it. My good friend Jen and I started e-mailing our daily food and workout habits back and forth to provide the accountability we needed. Two other friends joined us and the first "PEERtrainer group" was born.

One year later, I founded a Web site called PEERtrainer.com to help people who knew how to lose weight but had a tough time following through (like me). Since then, PEERtrainer has become the premier online weight-loss lab. The most well-known (and not-so-well-known) experts from every discipline approach us, write for us, and partner with us in order to deliver their most cutting-edge health information to our community. We bring this to the world every day. I see the problems and struggles people have with dieting on PEERtrainer, because I personally read every e-mail that comes in—and most of the struggles and problems are ones I have experienced, too. Our members share

> The only diet and exercise regimen that works is the one you'll actually do—a plan you'll follow through on.

feedback constantly. I know how people succeed, and what contributes to their failures. Through the resources at PEERtrainer, and the amazing PEERtrainer community, I've learned exactly what works and what doesn't. And what works is the Cheat System.

The foundation of *The Cheat System Diet* is the Cheat System. When we first created the Cheat System, it was just a simple list with very little explanation, a few recipes, and some gentle motivation. We didn't create a three-week plan. We didn't create a meal plan or an exercise plan.

We gave our members the basics because we wanted to see how the PEERtrainer community would respond—but also, more important, how our members would work with the list. Would they find it doable? Would they lose weight? What parts would they find confusing and what parts would they love?

More than 100,000 people downloaded our simple twenty-six-page PDF. After about a year, we surveyed our community to find out how they did with it. By just doing the basics, members had an average 14.2-pound weight loss over a three-month period. We learned not only was the Cheat System doable, it was also successful—and everyone was asking for a full plan. This book is that full plan.

The Cheat System is simple. It's a list of "Eats" (foods that will help you lose weight) and "Cheats" (foods that hinder weight loss). We take out complicated calculations, we convince you that starving yourself won't work, and we make it so food doesn't drive you crazy. You're no longer consumed by the thought of how you're going to get through a lunch with coworkers or "obligation" meals at your in-laws. The Cheat System builds on what you already know—that some foods are great for you, and others aren't—by giving you a super-easy way to think about eating, incorporating exercise, and enjoying life into your diet. We make it easy for you to lose weight without restricting a single food from your diet.

Some diet and exercise experts focus on the science of losing weight: nutrition, cortisol, hormones, etc. Others zero in on exercise. Some diets concentrate on every calorie you eat. Some focus on nutrients. Some emphasize on eliminating entire food groups. And though all of these factors have a hand in weight loss (and we'll go over the key points of each in this book), what's most important is *finding the plan that you'll do*—and that won't cause the same frustration most of us feel with old-fashioned diets.

With *The Cheat System Diet*, we reverse-engineered weight loss by focusing on the behaviors and habits you will actually follow through on, no matter what—even if your kids are in trouble at school or if your client is exceptionally demanding that day. We created a plan that people can actually do in real life, one they can follow through on.

When I was trying to lose weight myself, I became very angry at the way the world tries to help us lose weight. Most people I talk to don't need to be cut or have huge muscles (and if you are one of those people, inspired by growth hormone and testosterone-filled bodies, this book is not for you). Most of us don't want to sacrifice our time with our family or friends to hours in the gym. We just want to look good and feel good. We just want to go shopping and find a dress, pants or outfit that looks great—and not have to have to try on fifty different things, just to find something that fits. We want energy. We want health. We want not to be tired all the time.

Many diet and exercise plans are extremely regimented, but if you follow them to the letter, you'll have that perfect body. Because we don't necessarily want to sacrifice living our lives to become that perfect specimen of health and fitness, we can't follow those plans exactly, and we feel guilty or lazy. *The Cheat System Diet* lets you keep the foods you love, stops the guilt about your third glass of wine, and gives you a simple way to live your life.

I get that you're guilty about the wedge of cheese that you ate, the missed workouts, and your chocolate habit. I get that if you're a parent—especially if you're a mom—you sometimes feel like you're a slave to your family without any time to yourself.

We've all woken up on a Monday morning, thinking, "This is it, *today is the day I'm going to start*." And then your husband asks, "Hey babe, where are my keys?" and next thing you know, you're roped into a ten-minute search, everybody is running late, and there is no time for anything you wanted to do, whether it was an early-morning workout, making a healthy breakfast, or packing your lunch.

Or maybe your morning goes like this: you've set your alarm ten minutes early so you can at least have a quiet few minutes with yourself. But as soon as you wake up, your daughter wanders in and she wants her hair in pigtails and you can't find the rubber bands and the next thing you know, that ten minutes you tried to carve out for yourself is *gone*.

Most of the people who preach about "making health a priority" or harangue you to just "stick to your diet," or inform you that what you really need is to pay a personal trainer to get in shape have no idea what it's like to live in the real world. But I do, and so do our members at PEERtrainer. I know what it's like to want to lose weight, to feel like you're doing *everything* right but nothing is working.

I remember when I decided running was *the* answer. I bought a Garmin watch to track my time and distance and ran four miles every day. For four months! I watched the scale creep *up* by eight pounds, making every excuse in the book about my weight gain. I couldn't understand: I increased my workouts; I increased my movement and activity. Isn't this everything you're supposed to do? I couldn't even imagine why my weight was going up. At one point, I even thought the scale was broken!

Maybe you are the thirty-eight-year-old mom who was skinny in her twenties but can't get back to that weight, or the sixty-year-old woman who has the time to make healthy foods and eat a ton of vegetables but still doesn't see any success on the scale, or a forty-five-year-old father who is a vice president at his company and makes time to take care of his family, someone who understands exactly how to lose weight but just can't find time to do the workout. Or maybe you're the guy who woke up at thirty-five with a beer belly, suddenly thirty pounds overweight and with no idea how you got there. Or maybe you're the person who is doing everything "right" according to what you see on TV and read in the health magazines, but no matter what you do, the scale doesn't move. *The Cheat System Diet* is for all of you.

Since we started PEERtrainer, more than 60 million unique visitors have visited our sites. We've been featured on the cover of *People* and in a spread in *Good Housekeeping*. Dr. Oz has recommended PEERtrainer and we've had one of our members featured on *Good Morning America* for losing 100 pounds. We were even ranked as "Best in Support" by *U.S. News & World Report.*

Once health, nutrition, and fitness experts realized that PEERtrainer had a huge number of members that were eager to hear information about health, weight loss, and diet, they came out of the woodwork wanting to reach our members. Each wanted their voice amplified to our audience, because they knew we had figured out how to help people follow through.

In this book, you'll hear from those leading experts, people we've chosen to join us on PEERtrainer. These people are trusted advisers, whose messages we believe in, and whose science, research, and advice can help you. Many are our personal friends.

But the true power of the Cheat System comes from the many members of PEERtrainer who follow the plan. Our members share what works and what doesn't. In this book, you'll finally learn why you're doing "everything right" and still can't lose the weight. Our members share stories with PEERtrainers and with me that they wouldn't feel comfortable sharing with their husband or partner, friends, family members, even their doctor. Because members can be anonymous on PEERtrainer, they open up. We learn their fears, their struggles, and their obstacles to losing weight.

And we've put it all together into the Cheat System.

This is why the Cheat System works. And it works for life.

HERE'S HOW MONIKA FROM ATLANTA USED THE CHEAT SYSTEM

"I used this system as my wedding diet. I went from 142 pounds to 132 pounds and felt wonderful for my wedding day. I think this works because it allows you to eat food from most food groups and not feel hungry. I would highly recommend it. You honestly feel better doing this diet." —Monika V., Atlanta, Georgia

We'll explain why what you're doing now probably isn't working (or hasn't worked in the past) but also what will work: eating until you're satisfied, working out less, managing your stress better—while still allowing you to live your life and have a margarita at happy hour or attend your niece's birthday party and enjoy a slice of cake.

I've learned and seen that tiny steps in the right direction every day lead to huge, significant, permanent shifts in your body. Think of it like compound interest. Your money can start small, but then grow day by day into something that's gigantic and that can completely change your life.

After creating the Cheat System, I am proud to say that I lost all of my pregnancy weight and a little more. I'm five feet five inches and fluctuate between 119 and 123 pounds. I don't live in the gym, I still want and eat pizza when things get hard, and I'm more comfortable with my body now than I ever was at twenty.

YOUR SECRET WEAPON

Even though you are living with a ton of frustration, confusion, and hopelessness that any diet solution will truly work, you have a secret weapon. Your secret weapon is an open mind. People who succeed on the Cheat System Diet are open to ideas that challenge the status quo, ideas that are different than anything they've read or heard about before.

The Cheat System Diet gives people a clear direction, and it also gives people permission to *go at their own pace.* Often we are told that we have a "responsibility" to make dramatic changes or that we just need to "make health a priority." While these sentiments are well intended, and do sometimes trigger the change you're trying for, for most people our brains will resist this—often in a big way

According to Dr. Srini Pillay of the Harvard Medical School, our brains are built for slow and steady change. Says Dr. Pillay, "Habit is the king that rules the brain. New habits must be nurtured in a steady manner." We want you to move toward the way of eating that works, *at your own pace.* At PEERtrainer, we've learned that people *love* having freedom, especially when it comes to what they put on their plates.

That freedom paired with the plan that you can incorporate into your life helps rewire your brain over time—making change easier for you to follow through on.

Stop following all the diets you say you're going to do, knowing that you can't possibly do them in real life. Don't start the diet that makes you give up bread if you know that the second you do give up on bread, you'll want to eat an entire loaf. Stop counting every single crumb that goes in your mouth, and stop stressing out when you can't possibly know how much fiber is in your entrée at dinner. Stop making it hard on yourself.

The Cheat System is forgiving but most important, flexible. *Nothing* is off the table. Join our hundreds of thousands of members who have had success with understanding how to lose weight without beating yourself up, and who know that the Cheat System works. You can do this. You can lose the weight with the Cheat System. And you will!

PART ONE

Easy Is Better Than Hard

CHAPTER 1

How Cheating Will Help You *Finally* Succeed

Why You're Doing Everything "Right" but Nothing Is Working

Accept what is. Let go of what was. Have faith in what will be.
—SONIA RICOTTI

If you're like most people, you've read all the books, you know what you should be eating and doing, and you have a great deal of knowledge about diet and fitness, but you have a tough time following through. The diet and fitness world "helps" by giving us contradictory solutions, ridiculous gimmicks, and impossible standards—all of which are completely frustrating, counterproductive, and unsuccessful. What I hear from PEERtrainer members all the time is that they've tried a bunch of different diets but nothing works—or nothing works for long. Succeeding at weight loss involves a lot of factors, both physiological and psychological. If a diet doesn't take into consideration both—and most do not—that diet has set you up to fail. Period.

The Cheat System Diet helps you tackle all that has stopped you from losing weight in the past, and will help you at every level—food and exercise, your body and your brain—so you *will* succeed. We've done it with our PEERtrainer members and I've done it for myself.

Welcome to what works.

YOU HAVEN'T FAILED DIETS, DIETS HAVE FAILED *YOU*

There are a million fads out there: go clean, do Paleo, go vegan, go gluten-free, go whole foods, do whatever your best friend's sister is doing or what you see Jennifer Aniston talking about in a magazine—but then you don't have time to shop and cook and produce the latest braised fennel, blah blah blah . . .

Or you hear about a certain kind of yoga that Giada De Laurentiis does, and you think, "Maybe that's it!" But you are so stressed out about *getting* to that magical yoga class that it doesn't even seem worth it to you anymore.

Exercise programs that gain massive popularity in a flash like P90X or CrossFit are basically the same as trendy diets like Paleo: supposed magic-bullet solutions that in reality don't work for most of us. Could you succeed in the short term using them? Sure, but these programs are tough and restrictive, which most people can't maintain over the long term.

This is why so many people quit these fad diets and exercise programs over and over again. I did, too. I quit when it gets too rough on the treadmill. I quit sometimes when I'm just sick of eating healthy food and really want a slice of pizza. I'm sure you've done the same.

There is a biological reason we quit, why we give up when something we're trying to do becomes too hard. It's called *homeostasis*, and it applies to both your body and your mind. Your body wants to be in balance, and when it knows it's not—say, because you're killing yourself doing two CrossFit workouts a day, or spending the day at your desk starving on a calorie-restriction diet—it will do whatever it can to get back into homeostasis, the place it feels balanced.

> "One of those days where I wake up and go, 'It would be so cool to be a vegan. Gonna start today!' Then I fry bacon."
>
> —Tyra Banks

Because of that, I would argue that quitting is not always a bad thing. It means you have taken on too much, and your whole mind and body is shouting, "This is not going to work." And your body and mind are right.

Designed for people who have quit before, the

Cheat System promotes homeostasis. It makes your body happy, and it's doable. The trick is to keep your body in homeostasis. If it isn't in biological balance, your body and your mind rebel.

> "The Cheat System is better than strict Paleo, where I could not eat beans or sweet potatoes."
> —Jessica, Gahanna, Ohio

When we make a drastic change, it's hard for our body and mind to stay with that change, so most of the time it wants to overcompensate for what's missing. This is the reason why when you think, "Okay, today I'm giving up chocolate completely," all you can think about is having ten large chocolate bars. You might not have even thought about chocolate if you didn't declare such a drastic change. The Cheat System helps you make gradual, subtle changes so your body doesn't rebel. It makes small, good "deals" with your mind, so your body can get used to a new homeostasis. The Cheat System presents a new way of shedding pounds; your body says I can deal with this and you actually follow through.

I'm solely focused on what works. As I've mentioned, I've been obsessed—for eight years—with one question: What will you actually do? What will you follow through on? And the answer is the Cheat System. I wanted my plan to work whether you are an eighty-hour-workweek investment banker or a full-time wife and mother.

Just This Once . . .

The problem with restrictive diets is that it's really easy to fall off the wagon. And the second most people go the slightest bit off track, they use it as an excuse to go crazy for the rest of the day or even the rest of the week. You wake up on Monday morning and you want a fresh start . . . but then someone brings donuts to the office, or your car tire is flat, or your daughter forgot a permission slip. So you think, "Just this one morning I'm going to go to Starbucks and get my usual low-fat latte and an apple fritter, one last time." But by doing that, you set yourself up for a terrible lunch and dinner. You go out for Chinese with your coworkers for lunch and by dinner you figure it doesn't really matter, so Monday is a total loss. So then you decide, "I'm going to start Tuesday." And then Tuesday might go okay, but when you weigh yourself on Wednesday it still isn't be better and you've been doing this all week and you decide that it doesn't matter what you do. And you give up once again.

You're probably very successful at other areas of your life. Why has weight loss been such a struggle? Here's why: in other areas of your life, you probably don't set unrealistic goals. In other areas of your life, when surprises happen that you don't expect, you probably roll with it, or at least handle it as best you can. When you slip up or do something wrong, you might chastise yourself for a moment and then let it go. When life happens, you don't beat yourself up.

But when it comes to dieting . . . you do all of those things. You set unrealistic goals of sticking to a restrictive diet. When a surprise is tossed your way—like donuts in the office—you freak out. When you eat a donut and slip up, you beat yourself up and decide that all your previous effort was a waste. This thought process is one of the biggest reasons other diets have failed you.

The fact is, diets stress people out. Workouts stress people out. Life stresses people out. And all of those things are keeping you from losing the weight. We did the science, we did the research, we did the trial and error with our members on PEERtrainer. And what we've found, overwhelmingly, is that the pounds come off when the plan is easy, when it's doable, and when it doesn't stress out the body.

So *many* things go into your body being healthy, and what most people don't understand that is the stress it takes to get to the grocery store to shop for a restrictive diet (much less to eat on it) and to work out for hours a day counteracts all the work you are doing because the stress biologically gets in the way of your weight loss!

Stress Belly

Have you ever experienced a day when you were ravenous *all* day? You get up hungry, eat your "normal" breakfast, and feel like in order to be full, you literally need to eat three more. Perhaps you've eaten two eggs, spinach, and fruit, but you could eat another two plates of food and you're wanting a donut or something more than usual?

That's cortisol, and it may be one of the reasons you haven't been able to lose the weight. A snacky, can't-get-full feeling is almost always cortisol out of balance. It's obvious why this is bad: if you're never full, then you're always eating, and that will definitely not help you lose weight. I have those days, and before I knew what they were all about, I was beyond frustrated.

A huge part of why you haven't been able to lose the weight is because of a cortisol imbalance, a hormone activated when you are stressed (which for most of us is pretty constant). If you have a belly, that's cortisol. If you feel like screaming because you're always frustrated, that's cortisol. If you can't concentrate on healthy food or finding a way to exercise because you feel like you're being pulled from all sides, that's cortisol. A lot of people write off being stressed all the time as something that's just part of life or getting older or having kids—but it's not. Constant stress is often the result of a cortisol imbalance, and a cortisol imbalance can cause constant stress.

Cortisol can have an effect on your testosterone and estrogen levels, as well as on your entire body chemistry. If your cortisol is out of balance, it can have a domino effect on the rest of your hormones. Unfortunately, cortisol can be the catalyst for thyroid, estrogen, and an entire host of other hormonal issues.

I learned a lot about cortisol from Dr. Sara Gottfried, a Harvard-trained physician and bestselling author of *The Hormone Cure*. When cortisol is at high levels, it increases insulin resistance, which causes your body to store fat. Unfortunately for us, cortisol is also released when you feel psychologically stressed—like when you have to turn down a happy hour invitation because you've decided to start a new diet, for example.

Cortisol is natural and can be good for our body in many ways, but it is also a major factor to why people can't lose weight (and also why some of us carry more fat in our belly than anywhere else). If you feel like you're doing everything right but you're not losing weight, that's an indication that your cortisol is out of balance.

High levels of cortisol makes you look older, it's what's keeping the fat on your belly, and it's keeping you from being able to do what you used to be able to do when you felt like you had it together. It's keeping you from making the healthy decisions you need to make in order to lose weight.

When I discovered that cortisol was a huge factor in weight, I felt like I had uncovered a huge secret. I knew from my own experience that stress was a big presence in my life—not only did I feel stressed out by my life in general but also by just choosing to be on a diet!

So how do you know if your cortisol is out of balance? You can get a saliva test at your physician's office, and I highly encourage to you to do this. But we all know how much time and effort it can take just to schedule an appointment. So I have something easy for you to do right now. I want you to ask yourself a question—and really answer honestly.

Do you ever feel like you can't deal? Like you're so overwhelmed that anything you have to do makes you think, "How am I going to get this done?"

If you identified with this statement, you're not alone. As Dr. Sara has said in her book, many of us have issues with cortisol, and "All roads lead back to cortisol." So if you're stressed, overly emotional, or feel like your life is spiraling out of control, pay very close attention to your cortisol.

So what can you do about it? Often when I tell people about the effect cortisol has on their body and their weight, I often get a response like, "I'll deal with my cortisol when I have a minute, thanks!" And I get that—you are busy, life is full, and cortisol is an invisible problem that isn't calling for your attention, dinner, or a clean soccer uniform right now.

But cortisol is probably one of the major reasons diet hasn't worked for you in the past. Since a cortisol imbalance is responsible for a lot of that extra weight, we designed the Cheat System so it reduced cortisol at every level: in the food you eat, when you work out, when and how often you feel stressed. (You could have low cortisol issues as well, and cortisol levels are different depending on the time of day. The only way to be certain is to go to your phyisican, but for many of us, we have high cortisol at the wrong times and this keeps the weight on.)

This is one of the major ways the Cheat System is different from any other diet you've tried: *it takes care of balancing your cortisol levels and the other things that are holding you back without you having to even think about it.*

If you're on the Cheat System, the diet and exercise plan will stabilize your cortisol and reverse its effects on your body, mind, and your feeling of crazy stress—all at once.

It's Not About the Discipline

You might think the reason you haven't succeeded thus far is because you don't have willpower or the discipline to "do" a diet. But that's not true. For instance, let's say you are on a portion-control diet. Your family orders a pizza for dinner and you promise yourself you'll just eat one slice, but you end up eating three.

Most people blame not being able to control their portions on a lack of discipline, but that's not really true. The reason you can't resist that third piece of pizza is physiological. It has nothing to do with your mental discipline and everything to do with biology (more on that later). It's confusing because the majority of us have plenty of discipline elsewhere in our lives: we go to work on time, we keep to a household financial budget, we play by rules set before us. But we don't remember any of that discipline when we slip up on our diets. We are too busy blaming ourselves. We just end up thinking, "I want to lose weight *so* badly, what's wrong with *me* that I can't resist this slice of pizza?"

And that's a faulty question, because your willpower or discipline has very little to do with the fact that you ate the extra two slices of pizza—that was a physiological response to hunger. Your body needs micronutrients for fuel. It's really that simple. Pizza has an extremely low micronutrient profile. You're eating the pizza and your body is screaming out, saying, "Where are my micronutrients? I need selenium. I need manganese!" (Just to name a few.) So your body's response is, "If I eat more, I'll get my micronutrients," which leads you to continue to eat and eat while your body is actually starving for the type of fuel it needs to go.

But here's the worst part: you eat and eat and think, "Where is my discipline? I want to lose weight so badly but I just can't do it. Here I go again." But your brain translates "Where is my discipline?" and "I want to lose weight so badly" into "What's wrong with me?"

And your brain responds: "You're right. What *is* wrong with you?" Our brains are primed to solve problems, not to understand the nuance and context of every situation. So when it hears a question, it doesn't necessarily fill in the appropriate response (because your body was still hungry for micronutrients). Instead, it tries to "fix" what went wrong in the situation. But because your brain can't turn back time and stop you from eating the extra slices of pizza, it tries to "teach" you. It makes you feel guilty because it thinks that will make you stronger next time. (Which it won't, but as we discussed before, the brain is just doing what it thinks will solve the problem.)

Worse yet, as you continue asking your brain the question "What is wrong with me?" a psychological "stack" of problems begins to build up in your emotions. We start to stack all of our negative thoughts together. As psychologist Martin Seligman describes in his book *Learned Optimism*, the question "What's wrong with you that you ate three slices of pizza" turns into "What's wrong with you that you can't lose weight?" which then turns into 'What's wrong with you that you aren't as thin and stylish and perfect as the other moms at her school?" which turns into "What's wrong with you for not having the money to send your daughter to the horseback riding lessons all her friends are going to?" which turns into "What's wrong with you for not having a better job?"

When we're in a negative stacking mind-set, it's hard to see ourselves as anything other than our failures. We don't see a mom who cares about her daughter. We see a mom who can't lose weight, who can't afford the riding lessons, who doesn't look perfect, who doesn't have a great job, who *is* a failure at weight loss, at life in general. And for those of us who are struggling with our weight that mind-set leads to thoughts like: *I am a fat person. I am a loser. I am incapable of losing weight.*

STOP IT! Stop that thinking right now. You *can* lose weight and you *will* lose the weight. The Cheat System will show you how, and why all the discipline in the world couldn't have helped you.

Nice or Necessary?

Have you ever heard the story of the frog in warm water? If you put a frog in boiling water, he'll jump out. Instead, if you warm the water slowly, he will slowly die. You've got to create the "boiling" water in your life. You've got to create leverage. You've got to create your "must." Most of us say, "I want to lose twenty pounds," but it doesn't really happen until we get focused and have the leverage like an event where we feel like we *must* do it. A high school reunion is a great example. Many of us gain the leverage to lose weight when we know we're going to see peers from twenty years ago. The pain of not showing everyone what we could have been is *greater* than the pain of limiting Cheats and focusing on the Eats. So we do it. This is also why a diagnosis or a poor visit at the doctor's office can be so powerful. You finally have leverage to change your habits.

So where do you get the *must* from? As you saw above, it usually comes from having a great need or the thought of extreme pain if you don't do something. The pain of facing people from high school at your current weight or looking fat in the pictures on Facebook would have been greater than anything else happening before that weekend. Actors have their must. They're always thin; they won't get paid if they are not. And pain—seeing a picture of yourself, hiding from social interaction—is sometimes what pushes people to lose weight. Another powerful must is being faced with a potentially fatal disease like diabetes.

I've heard a lot of desperation and frustration from our members at PEERtrainer. And I've also seen how much creating and deciding upon your *must* can change your mind-set. Define your *need* to lose the weight. Define your why—*why* you want to lose the weight. Manufacture your *must* and change the game—putting you solidly on the path to success. You have nothing to lose but the weight that's been holding you back.

WHAT'S IN YOUR WAY (OTHER THAN THE WEIGHT?)

My mom once told me that relationships should have ease and a flow; they should not be painful. If you have a miserable time at dinner with an old friend and you're miserable most of the time you get together, you should question that relationship. If you have to beg for your boyfriend to spend time with you, it's probably not working. I've found that my mom's advice applies to diets, too.

When I'm eating and working out the Cheat System way, I know I'm going to lose weight. I'm confident of the end result. We will help you get confident, too. Losing weight on Cheat System will be so much easier than your path has been up to this point.

I suspect that having read the above, you are thinking, "You think weight loss is easy? You so don't know me or my life or what I'm going through!" But bear with me. When you obsess about something— whether it's about finding The One or worrying how your child is going to do at a sports tryout—you get in the way of the ease and flow that needs to happen in order for you to be successful. The best advice I've ever heard about dating is that when you want to fall in love, you shouldn't obsess over every phone call. You should make yourself busy, have your own interests, and then love will walk through the door. The same applies to children: when you care about your kids but don't obsess over how every little thing in life is going to affect them, your children learn to stand on their own.

The same applies to weight loss. Your obsession with weight loss is what's keeping you fat. I believe this with every fiber of my being.

 "I really like the Cheat System because it provides me an easy way to be accountable without being obsessive. It focuses on adding healthy foods that are beneficial to most people, yet gives you flexibility to make it your own." —Eileen, South Dakota

It is the ease and the flow that allows the right date to become a permanent relationship and allows parenting to transform a child into a functional adult. You're going to use the same principles with the Cheat System. It will give you ease and flow so you are not obsessed and beating yourself up the next time a brownie is calling your name. The Cheat System is about fitting into your life and getting rid of obsessiveness about losing weight.

Now you might be thinking, "Oh, she's just telling me to be positive, be positive, be positive." I'm not saying you should ignore the difficulty and just pretend everything is okay. Your frustrations are real and they are sabotaging you every day. It's about acknowledging them and moving on. Anthony Robbins uses this analogy often in his talks: "I'm not telling you to look out in the garden and say there are no weeds. I'm telling you to look out in the garden, see the weeds, and not say, 'Oh no, why are there weeds, why is this happening to me?' Instead, you'll go pull the weeds out and move on." That is what this book, and the Cheat System, will help you do.

We're going to pull out your weeds. And the first one I want to tug on is the belief that you have to do crazy things to lose weight. People have the idea that in order to lose weight, you have to eat lettuce and salads all day long, or foods you don't like, and oh, on top of that you have to work out thirty minutes to an hour every day, drink eight glasses of water, walk for four miles in the right shoes, and oh, P.S., your workout clothes have to be clean, you have to find a babysitter because you can't bring your kids, you need to spend the money for the gym and the right workout clothes or a trainer. . . .

When we think like this—and most of us do—we create what Dr. Pillay calls "brain chaos." Brain chaos is when there are so many signals and circuits lighting up in the brain that it can't make a decision. When the brain is experiencing chaos, we either do nothing about the situation or stress out by trying to do *everything*. When we encounter brain chaos as related to dieting, we either give up completely—"what's the use?"—or try to incorporate everything we've ever heard, which also results in quitting.

It's insanity to expect success when you are trying to do everything at once or when you give up completely. Neither is a clear path to your goal. However, when you ask your brain to do things that are easy for it to handle, you avoid brain chaos. We've created the Cheat System to do just that. It presents a set of rules that your brain can deal with, and doesn't ask you to do everything all at once.

What Do You, Personally, *Need* to Lose Weight?

Your answer to this question might be: *I have to have a babysitter.* Or, *I need a completely different way route from work, because the commute is long and I don't feel like eating healthy when I get home.* Whatever your need is, it's real and it's valid. You are smart, you are ambitious, you know what you want—and in order to succeed, we need to harness those talents and to figure out how to make these obstacles to not losing weight disappear (or at least, get out of your way).

If you can identify your "if only" statement(s) for not losing weight—"if only I had money for a personal chef," or "if only I had money for a personal trainer," or "if only I wasn't so busy I could get to the grocery store to get healthy food"—you'll start to see something very interesting. We all have *if only* thoughts, and the secret is, once you take care of one *if only*, a new one pops up.

The thing about *if only* is this: we believe that it's our "magic bullet" to losing weight. We believe it is the one thing holding us back from success. We all have *if only* reasons, but the reality is that to lose weight, **dealing with where you are right now is the magic bullet.** This doesn't mean you shouldn't have wants and desires—you should, and I expect you to—but getting out of your own way (and making your *if only* reason disappear) starts with accepting and tackling the right now.

The first step to fulfilling your dream is accepting, right now, what your situation is. Right now, I don't have more money, I don't have a personal chef, I don't have a babysitter. But given all of that, what *can* you do or change or try right now?

My *if only* was "If only my commute hadn't changed and I could go straight to the gym after work, then I would lose weight." And then my commute did change so I *could* go to the gym after work, but I still didn't go! I had to accept that just wishing something was going to change wasn't getting me anywhere. Once I accepted this, I was able to make real change and started walking to work, because it was something I could actually do.

Because You *Can* Lose Weight. And You *Will.*

Get ready for a sentence that will change your life. If you're reading this in public place, go to a bathroom or your car because I want you to say this life-changing miracle of a sentence with me. Say this out loud.

I am so frustrated with trying to lose weight. I'm so x%$@* frustrated!!!!

Say it a few times if it makes you feel better. See if it stops you from jumping on the stress treadmill where you constantly beat yourself up for being the size you are, eating the lunch you ate, drinking the wine you drank last night—you see where I'm going. Acknowledge what held you back and what's standing in your way now from losing the weight you want to lose. Now I'll begin giving you the tools with the Cheat System that will make weight loss suck *seem doable*— because you'll see results.

WHY THIS WILL WORK (WHEN EVERY OTHER DIET HASN'T)

If you haven't noticed already, the secret to Cheat System's success is that we don't just tackle food and exercise. We know, after working with our members at PEERtrainer, that successful weight loss isn't just getting the food and exercise right, it's about the psychology: believing that you can do it and matching your desires to your expectations. That's why this book promises to help you lose lots more weight than using the Cheat Sheet (the list of what to eat and what to avoid, most of the time) alone.

After introducing the Cheat Sheet to our members at PEERtrainer, we found that people really wanted a plan, so we wrote this book. Based on the Cheat Sheet alone, our members lost an average of 14.2 pounds over a period of three months.

"The Cheat System has been the *only* healthy eating plan that has ever worked for me! Not only has it enabled me to lose weight I never thought I would get rid of, it was so simple, and it worked from the first day.

"Please don't think it's just another diet; it isn't—it gets rid of cravings and it's simple and easy to follow. Please, please, give it a go—you won't regret it. After years of trying every diet out there, this was the answer to my prayers because it works! I only wish you were in the UK, because there are thousands of people over here who need your help, too!"   —Dawn G., United Kingdom

But *The Cheat System Diet* is bigger than the Cheat Sheet (which you can find a full version of online at http://www.peertrainer.com /cheattracker). The Cheat System attacks all the aspects holding you back from weight loss. Almost everything you read in these pages will sound counterintuitive. For example, in this chapter, we talked about how to get your mind set on success, rather than focusing on dieting and repeating the same expectation of failure. In Chapter 2, we'll explain how you don't have to worry about fat content or fiber. In Chapter 3, we'll discuss how you should slow down and shorten the length of your workouts—as well as get off the cycle of stress you've been riding.

And in Chapter 4, we'll show you how you can eat whatever you want (within reason)—all of which will help you lose the weight that you've been trying to get rid of.

Plus, if you ever find that you need help, want support from others on the same path, or simply have a question you'd like to ask me, you can visit PEERtrainer for even more answers. There's a section dedicated especially to readers of this book, but really the whole site is a tool you should use whenever you like.

"Every single 'FREE' e-mail and article I have ever received from the PEERtrainer Team have been the key to solving the great and frustrating mystery of weight loss . . . I owe my success to the entire PEERtrainer Team, and believe me, I get asked all the time 'What are you doing, you look fabulous!' The answer is simply to pass along your Web site address!"   —Deborah, Saskatchewan, Canada

Yes, I'm going to give you the plan. And yes, I'm going to give you tips and tricks and advice and directions. And yes, I'm going to give you the Cheat Sheet—Cheats and Eats—which is the key to the Cheat System Diet. The Cheat Sheet breaks down every food, spice, herb, and beverage out there into two categories: the Eats—of which you can eat as much as you want—and the Cheats—which you limit but don't have to eliminate from your diet, ever.

"I like the idea that nothing is truly off limits. I have a vicious sweet tooth and am a big carb addict. While I know carbs/sugar are the key to my weight gain, I know I can't just walk away from them and be happy. I like the idea that I can still acknowledge them as part of my diet.

"Just do the Cheat System. It's probably the easiest 'plan' I've ever seen. You can slowly add more and more healthy foods to your diet and slowly phase out the 'cheats,' at your own pace. I have *never* been successful for more than a couple days (if that) on a rigid system. I don't even bother with them. But this worked."
          —Dawn M., Springfield, Ohio

By having *unlimited* Eats, you'll never be hungry between meals because you'll feel full for hours longer than you do now. The Eats are full of micronutrients, which will make your body run more efficiently and reduce physiological stress. (That might sound like a minor thing, but it's really the catalyst to dropping fat fast.) You'll have more energy during the day, and sleep better at night.

You won't be white-knuckling it on this diet. There are more Eats that you can have unlimited portions of than there are Cheats. You won't be hungry, and you'll have plenty of energy to make good decisions, and to keep making them.

YOU CAN DO THIS DIET

The more you move *toward* healthy eating and habits and behaviors and psychology and the more you move *away* from what you've been doing (the dieting status quo of restrictive diets and long tedious workouts that everyone fails to lose weight on but still believes in), the more effective your weight loss is going to be.

I created the Cheat System to be a basic framework that leads to a gentle shift over time. It's a simple system that is easy to follow, one that doesn't lead to people feeling bad about themselves. And most important, it's a system that helps to promote better health long term.

But the key to why the Cheat System works, really, is the word "Cheat." What if you could cheat and actually lose weight, stay on track and improve your health? What if you could have your bacon and lose ten pounds, too? You can, on Cheat System.

HOW TO MAKE THE CHEAT SYSTEM WORK FOR YOU

Four things to keep in mind as you start the Cheat System:

1. It's critical to have a road map.

No matter how much you commit to doing the diet, you are going to encounter pitfalls, setbacks, and challenges. It is just a part of life. If you aren't prepared to deal with any of those things, though, then you'll find yourself dead in the water. There is always going to be temptation around you. There is always going to be an end-of-season soccer team party, the donuts in the kitchen at work, and the weekend barbecues with sausage, ribs, triple cream cheese spread, and nachos, the buffets and vacations.

So you have to have a road map that keeps you focused and on track when those temptations abound. You want to be able to enjoy them from time to time without going off the cliff. You have to have a way to build these types of events into your normal lifestyle or you will find yourself continually frustrated.

The Cheat System Diet gives you that road map. It'll show you a simple way to keep track of your consumption without having to deprive and starve yourself.

2. Willpower is not enough.

Relying on your own willpower or discipline, as we discussed earlier, isn't a realistic or effective long-term weight-loss strategy. It is almost always a story with an unhappy ending. If you're white-knuckling your eating, the tension will eventually become too much and you will overeat.

When you're hungry—which you are when you are on a restrictive diet—you simply can't be disciplined or have willpower. Your stress and your hunger and your hormones and your cortisol overwhelm your body.

In order to succeed, you need to be well fed and happy—which is what the Cheat System does. When you deprive yourself, food is always on your mind. When you're well fed with healthy, high-nutrient foods, you're not thinking about food. You're just living your life, and that's a good thing. That's where we will be taking you.

3. Be patient and persistent.

You have to break the cycle of beating yourself up. You will be successful, but it's going to require some patience and persistence. You can't start eating the Eats and two days later be discouraged and give up if the scale doesn't move. All that does is further cement you in the faulty belief that it's not possible for you. Rubbish.

You *can* do this, but you have to be smart about it. It's not an overnight process (nothing that gives you real and lasting results is). It may take a bit of time to build the habits you need to get you there, so take a deep breath . . . and now another . . . and one more . . . and smile and be easy on yourself. You need to treat yourself with at least compassion and understanding. Be easy on yourself and you'll get much further much quicker.

4. You don't have to be perfect to succeed, either.

As our partner and diet guru and great friend JJ Virgin always says, "Go for the B+, not the A+." Perfection is impossible, and so is being 100 percent on your diet all the time. But what *is* possible is being on the diet and doing what you should, eating what you should about 80 to 85 percent of the time: the B+. We have built imperfection into the Cheat System—we are all human, after all! And even without perfection, it really works.

 "The whole idea of cheating allowed me to succeed without being perfect. Don't get it into your head that it is impossible; instead, see that it can and will work if you make wise choices and stick with them . . ."
—Tom S., Florida

Before we get into the details of the diet in the next chapter, I want you to know that I've thrown a lot at you. I've explained how your brain works, I've explained that you need your *must*, and we will get into all of that later, but right now, I want you to just think about one thing that's tripping you up. I know you're probably thinking, Jackie, there are 150! But concentrate on one thing.

Is it the candy on your secretary's desk at work? Is it the playdate where the other mom is drinking chardonnay and you can't say no? Or is it date night? Or is it the fact that your husband or roommate can eat whatever he or she wants and not gain weight?

I want you to pick that one thing and I want you to give it up or avoid that habit for one day. You give up the candy in the office, or say no to the other mom, or suggest an at-home date night where you make your husband or roommate a healthy meal.

You will see the effect. You will see results, even if it's teeny-tiny. And you will teach your brain that it's a better deal *not* to do whatever it is that's been tripping you up.

Before you start the Cheat System, you have to know that what you do will have a result and that you believe you can do it. We're still a carrot-and-stick mentality at a certain point, so you want and need your brain to be on board. Your brain must think that the changes you're making are a better deal. And you have to figure out what your *must* is. Write it down and write down your goal now. Make the water boil and jump out. And jump in to your new life.

CHAPTER 2

Why You Lose When You Cheat and Eat

Stop Counting Calories/Fat/Fiber/Sugar/
Nutrients, Stop Eating Too Little, Stop
Obsessing—and Stop Going Up and
Down on the Scale

Maybe you wake up, excited to start your new morning regimen: egg whites, whole grain bread, just a bit of low-fat cream cheese for breakfast, and you diligently head to the gym and hit the treadmill for forty-five minutes—*every* day, all week. You make that yummy new whole-wheat pizza recipe (it's whole grain so you know it's good for you). You go to lunch with your coworkers and eat "bad" food only twice this week instead of four, and maybe one night you couldn't stop eating the cheese and crackers. You think you've done the best you can, but then you get on the scale you see not an ounce lost—or maybe you've even gained half of a pound. *Arggh.*

Or maybe you're the kind of person who reads all the latest health research, loves to make healthy recipes for your family, and basically consider yourself a nutrition expert at this point. You have an incredible smoothie you drink for breakfast that contains two bananas, chia seeds, half an avocado, cacao nips, almonds, vegan protein powder, fiber, and a pound of spinach. Your diet is all healthy right through dinner, with loads of seeds, nuts, beans, all vegan—everything that the shows and the articles say will help you lose weight. So you just don't get why the scale goes up one pound, down one pound, stays the same. All that work—and you're still ten pounds heavier than where you want to be.

Or maybe you're the kind of person who can't resist trying the latest greatest diet everyone is doing. On one diet you're avoiding all GMO foods, on another you're eating only organic, another one has you avoiding dairy and eggs. Every few months, you try something new based on the latest research. All your friends are doing it, and of course you have to try it, too, after reading the success story of the mom who looks amazing and lost fifty pounds on what she says is the easiest diet ever. You go at each diet with excitement, and actually succeed in losing a few pounds, maybe even five. But as soon as you can't do the regimen exactly, those pounds come back with a vengeance.

Or you've just said to yourself: "I'm not going to diet. I can eat as long as I work out." And though you don't make a change nutritionally (well, maybe you have a bit less of this and a little more of that, because you're burning more calories now, and need more carbs or protein or whatever), you are a madman at the gym. One night you can't resist a cheeseburger and a coke after a hard day and a long workout. You figure, "It can't do that much damage," but when you get on the scale the next day, your weight has gone up. Again.

Or maybe none of these scenarios rings true. You know what to do, and feel like you have a great deal of knowledge about how to lose weight and follow through, but you're just not doing it. You just don't feel like it. The motivation just isn't there. You feel like you'll have motivation again, someday—but not today. Not this month, and maybe not even this year.

DIET CONFUSION: WHY YOU CAN'T LOSE WEIGHT NOW

Whether you identified with one of the earlier examples or not, we all know that there are a million "right" diets that promise to work, and we all know—unfortunately, through experience—that most simply don't.

There is a huge and broad spectrum of diets out there for people to try. At one end, you have what we call the "traditional diet narrative": eating "healthy" foods like egg whites, whole grains, and low-fat mayo with canned tuna. That kind of diet really emphasizes portion control. And though it can work in your twenties, when you're still the perfect hormonal specimen and may be able to resist the second slice of pizza, it's nearly impossible to rely only on portion control or willpower after thirty-five. And some of us even find it difficult to stick to a portion-control diet even at a younger age.

There are also the only-vegetables-all-the-time diets and the elimination diets, which focus on eating lots of vegetables. The research linking increased micronutrient intake to health states and weight loss is overwhelming. No doctor will ever dispute an increase in eating vegetables. And many physicians agree that the elimination of certain foods has proven to decrease inflammation and to have positive benefits. However, people find the only-micronutrient plans and the elimination-of-entire-food-groups plans challenging because the diet seems restrictive and daunting. Most don't know where to start—and even those that do, end up finding these diets nearly impossible to follow through on.

It's important to note that all of these diets do "work"—but only if you can stick with them. If you are accurate at portion control and can restrict calories day in and day out, you can lose weight and maintain your weight loss. If you eat an entirely vegetable diet day in, day out, you will massively improve your health and you will lose the weight. If you permanently eliminate large categories of foods on an elimination diet, your inflammation will go down, and you will likely lose, weight.

But we've concluded, through observing hundreds of thousands of people on PEERtrainer, that weight loss on these diets tends to be temporary. Because who can eliminate large food groups—wheat, eggs, dairy, corn, sugar, peanut butter—every day for the rest of their lives? We've seen that though many people can do this for a period of time (though some people can't do it at all), most fail at maintaining such a strict regimen.

If you want to lose weight and keep it off, you must marry what is scientifically proven to work for weight loss with what is doable in your life right now. And that's the Cheat System.

In creating the Cheat System Diet, we reverse-engineered our diet plan. We knew a diet could work but that most people couldn't follow through. What we realized is this: the best information is recommended out of context. It doesn't take into consideration that we travel, that sometimes the only option is a convenience store or a fast-food restaurant. So we started with a new question: What would people actually do, day in and day out, in real life?

THE THREE ESSENTIAL PILLARS

There are three major pillars that put the best, most up-to-date and proven science of weight-loss information into the context of everyday life—marrying what works with what's actually doable.

1. High-Nutrient Eating
Eating foods with a high density of micronutrients—that is, green leafy vegetables—is the key to feeling full and improving health.

2. Limit Cheats
The ability to eat foods you still want, need, and crave—but keeping these foods a small part of your diet. A successful plan has to be flexible and forgiving enough to include social events where you'll have wine and dessert (and clear enough so that you understand exactly what and how much you are eating).

3. Reduce Inflammation and Shrink the Fat Storage System
The stress hormone cortisol and the inflammatory reaction from our immune system can work together to keep weight on (or even cause us to gain weight). Reducing our levels of cortisol help us slow this cycle, which not only prevents our body from adding more fat but also reduces inflammation overall, which helps burn more fat—accelerating weight loss.

Let's begin with the three essential pillars.

PILLAR 1: HIGH-NUTRIENT EATING

Micronutrients. Beans. Vegetables. Have your eyes glazed over yet? Wake up! *Wake up!!* It isn't enough for you to eat your vegetables be-cause everyone tells you to. You need to really know why you must eat them and the reasons have to be compelling—and they will be. (Dr. Joel Fuhrman, a partner of ours, explains this better than anyone I know. I'll introduce him in a moment.)

I have a question for you to consider. Why can't we stop at one slice of pizza? Why is portion control so hard? *Because you can't con-trol portion control when you are hungry.* Your hunger almost always takes over. You go in with good intent, thinking, "I'll just have one slice of cheese." Sometimes you can actually stop at one when you're focused, or when you have an event coming up and you have to lose the weight. But in real life, in everyday life? One slice becomes five—especially at night or after you've had a bad day. The reality is, after one piece of pizza, you're actually still hungry—for good reason. The typical portion-control strategies set you up to eat a restricted amount of very low-quality nutrient foods. One piece of pizza rarely fills you up because there are very few micronutrients in pizza, and only foods with a high micronutrient profile can curb your hunger. All the disci-pline in the world—the mantras like "nothing tastes as good as thin feels"—goes out the window when you're really hungry. And you're really hungry. And this is because the only thing that makes you feel full is high micronutrient eating.

MICRONUTRIENTS VERSUS MACRONUTRIENTS

All food has macronutrients (that is, proteins and fats), but some foods have higher micronutrient content (plant based phytochemicals) than other foods. Micronutrients are nutrients required by people in small quantities to orchestrate a range of physiological functions. Micronutrients give us the best fuel and, most important, help us feel full. Examples of micronutrients are calcium, copper, and manganese. Some of the most common foods we eat—like pizza and pasta—have a poor micronutrient profile, and the Eats have a high micronutrient profile.

On the Cheat System, you won't have to worry about the macronutrients, but remember that foods with lots of micronutrients are what makes us feel full.

The Best Diet Pill You Can Buy—At the Grocery Store

If we were to put a hundred doctors and diet experts in a room, everyone would disagree about the best way to help people lose weight. But the one thing all those experts would agree with is that eating vegetables and other high-nutrient foods is important. Incorporating more of these foods in your diet will help you drop pounds, increase your energy, and improve your overall health.

Vegetables are a *must*. Most people know veggies are good for them nutritionally, but can be harder to include in their meal, so they just think, "I'll do it next time." But here's the truth: Research has shown that simply increasing the amount of high-nutrient food in your diet is *more effective* for weight loss than controlling or decreasing portion sizes of any food. In fact, not only do people who eat high-nutrient foods tend to weigh less than people who eat more low-nutrient foods, **but they also eat more food.** You read that right. They eat a ton more food, but they weigh less. You may be thinking, how is that possible?

There are three reasons why.

1. All Calories Are Not Created Equal

Keep in mind that 100 calories of salad is totally different than eating 100 calories of an apple, potato chips, or SnackWell's. But here's what I want you to focus on, which comes back to the reason it's so hard to stop at one slice of pizza: If you choose the salad, you'll eat more food—and you'll be full longer.

High-micronutrient foods contain more fiber and water. Eating 100 calories of peppers, cucumbers, or spinach will make you feel fuller, for longer, than 100 calories of any so-called healthy food like brown rice or whole-wheat pasta. (More on that later.)

Our stomach digest foods with fiber slower than it digests anything processed. Your stomach digests a tablespoon of sugar in six minutes. A slice of whole-wheat bread? There's some fiber in that so you digest it in about twenty minutes. But kale? Hours. Unlike the bread or the sugar, your body has to work harder to digest the kale. And while you're digesting it, the high fiber content will keep you feeling full.

Before I go on to Pillar 2 . . .

I know what you're thinking: I'm telling you that eating vegetables is going to help you lose weight—and you're probably just thinking: I've heard this before! But I promise you, vegetables are going to be your new best friend. When you focus on Eats such as artichokes, salsa, and sweet potatoes, you'll not only be fuller for longer and have tons of energy but will make better decisions—all of which combines into weight loss.

Let me show you a simple diagram of three stomachs, used with permission from Dr. Joel Furhman's book *Eat to Live*. With over 1,200 references supporting high-nutrient foods and health, *Eat to Live* is the most well-structured argument out there for why vegetables are king for weight loss. The diagram below shows what your stomach looks like when it eats 400 calories each of fat (an oil), a protein (chicken), and Eats. (Joel used spinach, eggplant, and beans.)

Look at that! No wonder it's so hard to maintain the high-protein-and-nothing-else diets. Your stomach needs foooooood. It needs

MORE BULK MEANS FEWER CALORIES

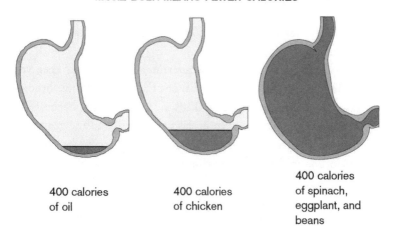

400 calories
of oil

400 calories
of chicken

400 calories
of spinach,
eggplant, and
beans

micronutrients. It wants to feel full. It doesn't care about "nothing tastes as good as thin feels"—because thin doesn't feel good.

2. The Best Little Fat Burners in the World

On the Cheat System, you can eat however much it takes of the Eats—which are all high micronutrient foods—that you need to feel satiated and full. You can eat as much as you want, no restrictions, because Eats are the key to your feeling full. How did we discover this "full" secret while everyone else is out there chanting willpower slogans while they're starving? Through Dr. Joel Fuhrman. Fred Nazem, health visionary, investor and founder and former chairman of Oxford Health, first introduced us to Dr. Furhman. After we read his books and research, it was impossible to go back. In *Eat to Live*, Dr. Joel Fuhrman proves that even if you eat more volume (a bigger amount) of high-micronutrient foods than you would of low-micronutrient foods, you end up eating fewer calories. Fuhrman's program is based on the acronym G-BOMBS (greens, beans, onions, mushrooms, berries, and seeds) because these foods have the most powerful anti-fat storage effects and the highest level of micronutrients. Consider kale (or spinach or greens) versus brown rice. If you eat 100 calories of kale, you've eaten about 3 cups of kale—versus 100 calories of brown rice, where you've eaten about ½ cup (cooked). (If you were to eat 100 calories of pizza, that would be half a typical slice.) You may have eaten the same amount of calories, but the kale gives you more bang for your buck—and you will feel full!

And here is where it gets interesting: Eats not only keep you feeling full, they help you burn fat. The Eats, especially mushrooms (always make sure they're cooked), function as "angiogenesis inhibitors." Angiogenesis is a process that results in the growth of new blood vessels from pre-existing vessels. In cancer, for example, angiogenesis occurs when a tumor grows large enough to need its own blood supply.

What's interesting is that the growth of fat tissue is dependent on this exact same process. When you increase the amount of high-nutrient foods, especially broccoli, mushrooms, onions, greens, and berries, you are eating a diet that fights angiogenesis, making it hard for fat to get its own blood supply and grow.

Researchers are starting to look into what they call "pharmacological manipulation of adipose (body fat) tissue (to) offer a novel therapeutic option for the treatment of obesity and related metabolic disorders." Translated into English, that means that drug companies are trying to turn the properties of these foods into drugs. But you don't need that—you just need to eat the Eats in order to give your body the same results: losing weight.

BROWN RICE VERSUS WHITE RICE—GUESS WHAT, IT'S IRRELEVANT!

So I mentioned earlier that kale will make you feel more full and help you lose weight more than the so-called healthy brown rice or pasta. And I'm about to make a totally controversial statement. Eat white rice over brown rice if you love it. The brown rice versus white rice debate is irrelevant. Why in the world would I say, it's irrelevant when you're always being told to that brown rice is the better option over white rice?

The debate is irrelevant because there's very little difference between the micronutrient profile of brown rice and the micronutrient profile of white rice. Years ago, Dr. Joel Fuhrman developed a system that ranks foods according to what they contain that's good for our body, including vitamins, minerals, and as many known beneficial phytochemicals as possible. He calls this the ANDI scale, and each food has its own ANDI score, which is actually the basis of all those numbers you see above products in Whole Foods.

Dr. Furhman's scale ranges from 1 to 1,000, with 1,000 being the most nutrient dense. You can guess that kale is at a 1,000. So are mustard greens. Other vegetables that come in well above most other foods include spinach (707), arugula (604), romaine lettuce (510), carrots (458), Brussels sprouts (490), and broccoli (340). Berries also score relatively high, with strawberries leading at 182 and blueberries in second place at 132.

But "healthy" brown rice? A paltry score of 28. And white rice? Its score is 12. There is only a 16-point difference between brown and white rice on a scale that ranges from 1 to a 1000. And by the way, French fries are 12, too. It's clear that in terms of nutrition, vegetables are better choices, in terms of eating for nutrition, than any of these foods. So if you want white rice? Eat it. Both brown rice and white rice are low on the ANDI scale. They won't make you feel full. Remember, the high-nutrient foods are king.

3. No More Hunger or Toxic Withdrawal

I was with a family member a few months ago at lunchtime, and we both made salads for ourselves. I made a huge salad and filled a large bowl, similar in size to a family salad bowl. She made a salad about one-third the size of mine and placed it on a square appetizer-size dish. So we ate: my salad in this huge bowl, and hers on this little dish. We had nearly identical salads, but we had completely different portion sizes.

When we were both done eating, she said that she was still hungry; she actually said, "I'm starving."

I responded, "Of course you're still hungry! Who wouldn't be starving on that little tiny dish of salad?"

"You ate a pretty big bowl, didn't you?" she replied. I told her that I always eat out of a big family-sized-bowl or order at least two or three vegetables sides at a restaurant, because that's what keeps me from being hungry.

She responded, "Do you think I could make and eat another salad and still lose weight?"

The answer is yes. YES! YES! YES! Vegetables are the best diet pill in the grocery store. I told her to go out that day and buy two *large* salad bowls. Why two? Because if you have two, then one will almost always be clean.

The truth is, most of us don't eat enough high-nutrient foods (Eats) to not feel hungry. But on the Cheat System, you will—your body will get what it needs to feel full, even between meals.

A study published in 2010 *Nutrition Journal* showed how people who ate low-nutrient dense foods tended to be hungrier more often than people with high-nutrient dense diets. That may be why, when you eat a sandwich for lunch, you end up craving a latte and a scone just a few hours later.

Interestingly, the researchers hypothesized that one of the reasons why the people in the study had less hunger on a high-nutrient diet is because a low nutrient-dense diet can cause "toxic hunger," hunger that wasn't true hunger but rather was caused by metabolic dysfunction. Increasing nutrient density reduces the feeling of toxic hunger, making the sensation of hunger much more tolerable.

While eating a diet high in vegetables and fruits, your body simply doesn't have the same hormonal reactions as it would on a portion-controlled only diet. Your blood sugar and insulin are relatively stable, and your body doesn't freak out about having enough food to fuel itself. You feel full, and because you're eating enough during the day, you don't dive into the cheese and crackers every night. That said, we still want to be able to have cheese and crackers. We can't only eat high-nutrient foods 100 percent of the time. Well, most of us can't. Which is why the Cheat System works. You feel full from your Eats, but you still have your Cheats. Like a glass of wine. Or whatever you need to feel satisfied.

ARE YOU "GOOD" ALL DAY BUT "MESS UP" AT NIGHT?

For years at PEERtrainer we have seen a phenomenon in which people feel as if they do great all day and then "mess up" at night. We've figured out why this happens—and the solution is right here in this chapter. The reason that you find it impossible to resist the cheese in the fridge and the crackers in the pantry is because you're not eating enough high micronutrient food during the day. This is why in the Cheat System Diet, many foods are *unlimited*. If you're full at breakfast, lunch, and dinner, you'll be able to say no to the cheese at night—because your body will have had everything it needs for the day.

There is so much pushing against you from succeeding when you diet. Most of the time, you're not getting the emotional, physical, or nutritional support your body needs to operate at its best. But the Cheat System will provide your body with the physical and nutritional resources it needs to lose weight—and curb the late-night trips to the fridge that are holding you back now.

On the Cheat System you're going to feel full. Because you're going to be eating *unlimited* amounts of Eats. We're going to show you how to do it—you're not going to have to white-knuckle it through the evening anymore after a really hard day. And when you're at a party, you're still going to be able to eat cheese. You're still going to be able to have chocolate. That's where the second pillar comes in. . . .

PILLAR 2: LIMIT CHEATS

To make anything stick for the long term, you're going to have to be able to live in the "real world." You're going to have to be able to go to a party and not stress out about food. This is where the second pillar comes in—being able to eat foods you love, but with the plan of knowing your Cheats. When you know your Cheat limit, you can still have Cheats and lose weight. This is all about the delicious Cheats.

This is not about eliminating foods or counting and figuring out every single calorie, fiber, and fat, and measuring everything you eat, because both of those things are untenable. There will always be a day you're stressed out and you go off track. You still have to eat at your mother-in-law's, your friends will still want to try the amazing new bakery, and you will want a cupcake. But most important, if you try to do a portion-control-only diet, you'll almost always be wrong: you'll almost always be eating more than you think.

How does portion distortion happen? It can happen when you start to date someone new or get married, or when you see your partner eat a ton more than you. Suddenly your idea of portions get skewed. Or maybe when you were pregnant your hormones went out of control and you ate everything in sight. And now you're post-pregnancy, and after nine months, it's hard to eyeball what a "reasonable" portion is anymore. And additionally, you find yourself obsessing about food.

In a 1993 study published in the *New England Journal of Medicine*, which was later repeated and proven by similar studies, researchers asked participants to record their calories. The researchers then compared what the participants said they ate to what they actually ate. The participants underreported their daily average intake by 47 percent! That would be the real-world equivalent of eating 147 calories, while thinking that you only ate 100. If you were following a calorie-counting/portion-control-only diet, at 1,700 calories in a day, you could be eating 799 more calories a day! That's almost 800 calories more—2,500 calories a day in reality versus what you are thinking you're eating: a 1,700-calorie-a-day diet. And that's 3,500 more calories per week. You can just imagine what can happen after a month and a year. No wonder portion control fails so many people.

Why Portion Control Failure Is Not Your Fault

Even when people are taught accurate portions, they can't keep to their diet. In two different studies, done years apart, researchers tested how well people gauge proper portions and each time got the same result. In both studies, the researchers divided participants into four groups. Each group was taught proper portions: how much and what to eat. Three groups were given meals with correct portions measured for them and the fourth group had to make their own meal after just learning proper portions. I'm sure you can guess what happened. The groups who were given the meals lost more weight than the group who had to make the meal themselves. They were all taught proper portion control. They just couldn't do it on their own.

There's also a psychological component. In a different experiment, researchers asked participants to eat a bowl of soup that was supposedly the "right" portion size. But what the participants didn't know was that one bowl was normal and the other was bottomless.

When comparing the two groups after the study, researchers found that the people who had the bottomless bowl ate more. But here's the kicker: the people who ate out of the bottomless bowl didn't feel any more satiated than the group that had eaten the standard portion in the normal bowl. What the scientists concluded in that study was that perhaps visual cues—what size portions we see on our plate—affect our hunger and feeling full more than what we *actually* eat.

Portion control works, to some extent—which is why on the Cheat System, you'll count the Cheats you eat. What we learned from our PEERtrainer members is that portion control works if you have a lot of forgiveness built in. That's why we make it a part of the Cheat System. You can have bacon—one medium slice of cooked bacon is one Cheat—but you'll be coupling those calories with feeling full and lots of micronutrients, not depending on the bacon alone to fill you up. When you count your Cheats and eat your Eats, you'll be able to lose weight and still go to a dinner party. And you can have some ice cream when you're really stressed. Because these Cheats are part of the plan—they won't destroy your entire weight-loss strategy.

PILLAR 3: REDUCE INFLAMMATION AND SHRINK THE FAT STORAGE SYSTEM

In Chapter 1, we discussed how cortisol might be the reason you haven't been able to lose the weight. There are two other major biological factors that impact weight, both how much we lose and how much we gain: inflammation and hormones. The Cheat System tackles both head-on, without you even having to think about it.

Inflammation: The Biggest Weight-Loss Inhibitor

Inflammation is a reaction from our immune system. Acute inflammation is obvious—you stub your toe, it swells for a while and then goes back to normal. When the injury is healed, acute inflammation is gone. Chronic inflammation, on the other hand, can be pretty covert: it can be present in the body for a long time without being visible or noticeable in any way. Anyone —and I mean anyone—who is even a few pounds overweight has chronic inflammation. And chronic inflammation keeps the weight on.

Performance nutrition expert Brian Rigby explains that scientists and doctors used to think that our fat cells were just a place where we stored excess energy. They now know that our fat cells are their own organ, just like our kidneys or our brain. And because our fat cells are their own organ, they produce their own hormones and their own inflammatory hormones. So when someone develops an excess amount of fat, that person ends up releasing hormones that cause more inflammation. This creates a self-perpetuating cycle: more inflammation, more fat, more inflammation, more fat, even more inflammation. . . . You get the picture.

Unfortunately, any extra fat stores—essentially even an ounce more than your body thinks you should have—leads to a state of mild, chronic inflammation. So how can we eliminate that inflammation for good, and get off the fat-inflammation cycle?

By eating foods that decrease inflammation. Foods rich in micronutrients and phytochemicals—the Eats of the Cheat System—decrease your levels of cortisol, tackling the problem head-on. Stabilizing your cortisol slows the fat-inflammation cycle and eventually reduces inflammation. Eats do all of that—and by decreasing inflammation, we're fighting the source! Your body will start acting in a more normal, healthier way.

Decreasing the inflammation in your body is the key to unlocking weight loss—because if you get rid of inflammation, you get rid of fat.

Not all fat is inflamed, and we do need some fat to survive. But if you are overweight, there's a good chance that your excess fat is inflamed; if you decrease that inflammation you will lose that fat.

The Fat Storage System: Hormones

We all know how hard it can be to lose weight after thirty-five. Dr. Sara Gottfried, an expert in hormones and the bestselling author of *The Hormone Cure*, told me why. Apparently we are the perfect hormonal specimen at the age of twenty-eight. After twenty-eight, your hormones start to change. If you're having trouble losing weight, your imbalanced hormones may be the problem. And guess what. Cortisol is a hormone. That's right. Cortisol—the thing that's keeping the belly fat on—is a hormone. As Dr. Sara says, it's one of the Charlie's Angels. Right alongside cortisol are the two other Angels: thyroid and estrogen. She calls them Charlie's Angels because these three hormones protect our body.

But when one of the Angels is compromised, it begins to compromise the power of the other two. Typically, the most common Angel compromised is cortisol, and this ends up affecting the thyroid and estrogen. That's why the Eats on the Cheat System are natural cortisol regulators. If you find yourself with excess belly fat or people are asking if you're pregnant, you most likely have an issue with high cortisol. (Of course, you should go get your hormones, including cortisol, checked with your doctor. There are times when your cortisol should be higher, namely in the morning. It's the high cortisol at night—the one that keeps you from falling asleep or wakes you up in the middle of the night—that's also the one that's keeping your belly fat.) When you're eating the Eats from the Cheat System, Eats attack high cortisol head-on—which really moves the needle when it comes to weight loss.

In addition to Dr. Sara's Charlie's Angels, there are a bunch of hormones out there that can be affected by good behavior. There are a whole set of hormones that are affected by sleeping better, by eating more nutritiously, and by managing your stress that makes weight loss easier. We'll explain more about how hormones work in your body in the next chapter, but for now, just know that the Cheat System will do the work for you when it comes to getting your hormones back in balance. Another way to reduce your cortisol levels and achieve hormonal balance? An elimination diet.

Elimination Diets and Hormonal Balance

Elimination diets encourage cutting out entire food groups like dairy, wheat, processed foods, GMOs, sugar, etc., the food groups shown to promote weight-loss resistance. And they work because they reduce intake of highly inflammatory foods.

Unfortunately, because these diets and cleanses restrict you from eating *so* many food groups, they're really hard to stick to when you go out with friends or to a party. It becomes so frustrating to try to find something to eat. An elimination diet, after a few weeks, becomes socially isolating and totally frustrating—you can't eat anything, ever!

That being said, doing an elimination diet can help you find out if you have any food sensitivities that could be holding you back from losing weight. Food sensitivities are totally real. Our good friend JJ Virgin, the bestselling author of *The Virgin Diet*, says that doing a cleanse helps you fall on a continuum. If you think you have a sensitivity, it can be a good thing to do a cleanse, so you can test out your theory.

But most of what you'll eat on the Cheat System (what we call the Eats) are not foods that cause intolerances and insensitivities. And because the foods that do cause those sensitivities will no longer be the center of your meal, the shift focuses to the high-nutrient, inflammation- and cortisol-fighting foods, which is where your focus should be.

WHAT DOES WORK: DIET FUSION (NOT *CON*FUSION!)

By combining the results of research studies done on weight loss and observing what worked at PEERtrainer, we realized that the diets at the polar end of the spectrum (and some in the middle) do work to some extent. Portion control works, up to a point. The elimination diets reduce inflammation and help you lose weight, but almost everyone trips up at a party or breaks down one night and binges on cheese. And while the radically healthy diets like Fuhrman's, which rely on eating tons of vegetables, feed you the nutrients your body needs and helps you lose weight, the restrictiveness of a super-healthy diet like that is difficult to maintain outside of your own kitchen.

What the diet world needs is something that takes the best ideas and brings them together in a plan that really works. This is exactly what the Cheat System does. We call this concept *diet fusion*, and it's the foundation of the Cheat System Diet. We understand that nutrient-rich foods, including vegetables—what we call Eats—are king, while at the same time acknowledging that we live in the real world and are going to have a cookie or enjoy a cheese plate at a party.

The Cheat System is common sense. You eat healthy most of the time, so it's okay to indulge yourself every once in a while. You'll eat well 80 percent of the time, so the other 20 percent doesn't matter nearly as much as if you ate that food all the time.

Plus, the Cheat System is designed to be easy. A lot of people try and fail on diets that require you to count the calories in everything you eat, or figure out how much fat and fiber were in your foods—because that's tough to do at every meal, especially when you have to eat outside your own kitchen.

On the Cheat System, you don't have to do any of that. We've

figured out the nutrition for you. We've divided foods into two different categories: the Eats and the Cheats. This is the marriage between
what works and what's actually doable, and it's what will help you lose
the weight.

WHY CHEATING AND EATING WORKS

The Cheat System has you eating the same way that studies have
shown lower caloric intake overall, reduce hunger and cravings, and
increase the level of satiety at every meal. And while portion control
has been shown over and over again in scientific studies *not* to work
unless you are served preportioned meals in a controlled environment
or plan to eat all pre-packaged meals, there have been studies that
show how people who eat a **diet with a foundation similar to the
Cheat System diet lose three times as much weight as people who
rely on portion control alone.**

In fact, some of the most successful, clinically studied diets, including one featured in the journal *Nutrition Reviews* in 2001, use the
exact same approach as the Cheat System: eating foods that are good
for your body with small amounts of Cheats.

Eat the Eats, but Count Your Cheats

The mistake many of us make when we're busy and just trying to get
things done is that we don't think our food choices through. We think,
"Oh, just this one time couldn't hurt." But it's never just one time. One
time leads to another one time, and then it's multiple times, which end
up stacking up into pounds gained. I remember the day I discovered
the Salted Caramel Hot Chocolate at Starbucks. I said, "Okay, I'm just
going to get a small." Well, I did that every day for a month.

One day I thought, "What's really in this thing?" So I asked. The
barista started reading the ingredients and I couldn't believe what I
was actually drinking! The signature drink was around three cheats,
and that was without the whipped cream.

We are all going to make mistakes, including me. And you're probably going to make those mistakes more often than you like. But the best thing about Cheat System is that you're able to make mistakes. You don't need to be perfect, because the Cheat System is designed for that. When you eat a truly healthy diet most of the time, eating Cheats won't harm you as much as it would a person who *only or mostly* eats those foods.

Imagine a scale, the kind with two sides that balance out if left empty. The Cheat System is like that scale: as time goes on, you will realize that by choosing to eat mostly Eats, you will have more energy, lose more weight, and make better choices.

Cheating + Eating = Energy

Every meal on the Cheat System will provide you with enough energy to sustain you through the day. You may find that you feel more energy than you have in years. That's because a typical meal on the Cheat System has everything your body needs to function—without the rush/crash/rush cycle that sugar and caffeine have.

One of the most important lessons we learned from our PEERtrainer members is that you have to have energy to make good decisions, and that your weight loss really hinges on what kind of decisions you make. Most decisions that really affect weight loss seem simple: I'm going to have a salad with chicken at lunch, or I'm going to have the pasta. You simply choose the healthy choice or the not-healthy or less-healthy choice. With each decision, you are making a deal with your brain; for every small choice you make, your brain has to feel like you're making the better choice.

For instance, let's talk about French fries. If I had to pick America's number one indulgence, it would have to be French fries. Once you tell yourself you can never eat French fries, your brain goes "Wait, that's not a great deal!"—so it starts freaking out. However, since you can eat anything you want (including French fries) on the Cheat System, if you decide to pass on French fries at lunch, your brain says, "Oh, no problem, I can eat French fries another time. I can do that."

DRINK WATER!

Consuming water is the best, most important thing you can do for your body—and for weight loss. Our body is mostly composed of water—because nearly everything needs it, from cells in our organs to our blood and our brain. When you don't drink enough water, your body simply doesn't perform the way it should. Without enough water, your muscles may even be weaker, making any workout or physical activity you do less productive.

You should try to drink half your body weight in ounces every day. So, because I weigh around 120 pounds give or take, I should drink about 60 ounces of water—roughly eight 8-ounce glasses of water—each day. If you don't like the taste of water for whatever reason, feel free to naturally flavor it with berries, grapefruit, lemon, or cucumber (which are Eats . . .).

WHAT CHEATING AND EATING LOOKS LIKE ON A PLATE

A Cheat System meal combines healthy fats, traditional protein, and Eats to provide all the energy you need for the day. These three things should always be on your plate. I understand that I said "always," but this is ideal. If you can't, you can't—don't let that stress you out and drive up your cortisol.

1. Healthy Fats

Healthy fats are essential. Without them, you wouldn't be able to live. Healthy fats include omega-3 fatty acids (found in fish, fish oil, chia, and flax seeds) and monounsaturated fats like olive oil, all of which have positive effects on our blood. Almonds and avocados are also natural, healthy fats. Healthy fats also include the triglycerides found in coconut oil and goat milk, which have a unique biochemistry that prevents them from being stored in the body. Instead, they are burned for energy right away.

If you eat fat—no matter what kind—it will enter your blood. Eating a lot of "bad" fats can cause atherosclerosis (fat deposits in your arteries) and other health problems, but "good" fats help the good cholesterol in your blood and are great for your heart. So, in addition to making food taste better, eating healthy fats keeps you healthy.

Healthy fats also make us feel satiated. When you add a good fat to a meal, it will not only make the dish more tasty but it will also send the same signals throughout your body that provide the satisfaction and satiation factor that unhealthy fatty foods do.

And your first serving of the day of healthy fat is Cheat free!

SALT SUGAR FAT

In the popular book by Michael Moss, he shows how food scientists have worked very hard to create the right amount of sugar, salt, and fat in processed foods so that people will keep eating. The right combination of these will create the satiation point: where the food is flavorful, but bland enough to keep eating—like the perfect potato chips. A meal that is greater or lower than this point will not have this same effect.

No physician or nutritionist will dispute that large amounts of sugar is bad. Most people know that eating sugar adds calories, and it does. But the bigger issue is that sugar can cause the same reactions in your brain as cocaine. Once you have some, you will always want more. That's why we consider processed and sugary foods "Cheats."

Most people eat way, way too much sugar. It's in almost every food on the planet, from Kraft Macaroni and Cheese (7 grams per serving) to apples (an average of 15 to 17 grams per apple). The problem isn't necessarily with the sugar itself, but that we're eating way, way, way too much—and it's not only making us fat but also making us really sick.

When you eat a meal, your blood sugar will naturally rise and a hormone called insulin goes to work at lowering your blood sugar. But when you eat a meal or a snack or a drink containing a lot of sugar, your blood sugar becomes really high. And that forces insulin to work overtime. (What most people call a sugar rush is having high blood sugar; the crash you get after binging on sugar is insulin doing its job and removing that sugar from your blood, resulting in you having low blood sugar.)

Typically, insulin moves the sugar from your blood to other areas of the body that need it, including your muscles, your liver, and your fat. If you eat excess sugar, your insulin will still have sugar left to store—which it puts into your fat stores. Over time, that excess sugar becomes extra weight.

When we eat something that is composed mostly of simple carbohydrates, like pasta, rice, or candy, our blood sugar rises rapidly. Suddenly insulin will rise to match it and dissipate the excess sugar to areas that need it and then to fat cells. But if insulin does that job really well—which it typically does—we end up feeling hungry again almost right away. When there is too much sugar in your diet, it's very, very easy to overeat, and not realize it.

But once sugar in the diet is limited, the body adjusts. It begins to use fuel from what already exists in the body. If you are relatively sedentary during the day—like most of us who have desk jobs are—the glycogen (the carbohydrate your body stores as fuel) in your liver will last about four to five hours without eating. Your body will adjust to burning extra fat between meals instead of expecting a snack or a meal to fuel itself every few hours, so the feeling that you're hungry all the time will slowly fade as your body makes those adjustments. It's just another way that eating the Eats causes us to be less hungry than eating any other way.

2. Traditional Animal Protein or Pea/Rice or Pea/Potato Protein

"Traditional" animal protein means meat, fish, eggs, or animal protein, and pea/rice or pea/potato protein means the protein powder used in PEERtrainer Cheat System shakes. We want you to have either have animal protein or a plant-based protein like pea/rice or pea/potato in your meal. (Again, this is an ideal—if it's impossible, do the best you can.)

You should know it's difficult to eat enough protein on a vegan or vegetarian diet to promote weight loss. It's not impossible, but it is difficult. If you're "going vegan" or eliminating traditional animal proteins from your meals in an attempt to lose weight, studies published in the *New England Journal of Medicine*, the *Journal of Cardiovascular Nursing*, and *Nutrition* have all supported that you won't be nearly as successful in dropping pounds as someone who incorporates "traditional" protein at every meal.

Drinking a breakfast smoothie made from plant-based protein kick-starts your day's fat burning by balancing blood sugar or insulin levels. A study in the *American Journal of Clinical Nutrition* showed a high-protein breakfast reduced ghrelin—a hormone that tells your brain to eat—better than a high-carb breakfast did. Lower ghrelin, coupled with a balanced blood sugar level, mean you're far less likely to make that mid-morning bagel cart or snack-machine trip.

That's why, on Cheat System, we ask for you to eat 4 ounces of traditional lean animal protein, such as chicken, fish, beef or an egg, or a serving of pea/rice or pea/potato protein from a quality source with every meal. And like the healthy fat, 4 ounces of traditional protein or one serving of the pea/rice or pea/potato protein at your first meal is also Cheat free!

WHY DO WE ADVOCATE FOR TRADITIONAL PROTEIN OR PLANT-BASED PROTEIN LIKE PEA/RICE?

These kinds of protein will keep you satiated. If you were to eat large portions of vegetables without traditional or pea proteins, you eventually would be satiated (remember those three stomachs). But most people don't eat enough vegetables to reach that point. You would have to eat two or three entrée portions of salads and vegetables to reach that point, for a typical 130-pound woman. Most people aren't willing to do that. Remember, I'm obsessed with follow-through, and for many people, it's just too hard to eat enough vegetables, without traditional protein, to feel satiated. So this is why we advocate a traditional protein.

The best part? If it's a PEERtrainer Cheat System shake, you can actually earn a Cheat for the day!

What Kinds of Traditional Protein Should You Eat?

Beef

There are significant nutritional differences in your beef choice depending on how meat is raised. Grass-fed is always the better choice.

Conventionally raised beef has much more fat than grass-fed beef—almost 2.5 times as much! If you're thinking, "But I trim the fat off my steak anyway," and while that's great to do, it doesn't really solve the problem. Conventionally raised cattle mostly eat grain like corn, which results in their muscles being marbled and makes for a tasty steak, but because the fat is intertwined with the muscle, it is impossible to "trim" this kind of fat from a cut of meat.

Grass-fed beef also has more healthy fats (for example, omega-3s) than traditionally raised beef. Omega-3s are cheap calories: omega-3s are used for maintaining and building cell membranes. They don't get stored as fat. (The only people known by researchers to actually store significant amounts of omega-3 calories as fat are the Inuit, who eat a fish-based diet. They consume so many omega-3s, they are basically forced to store some, but even they store only about 1 percent of what they eat.)

Brian Rigby also reminds us that grass-fed beef is also higher in two other healthy fats called conjugated linoleic acid and vaccenic acid, which have been shown in research to potentially increase our body's ability to burn fat.

So go grass-fed when you can, but don't stress about it. If you can't afford or find grass-fed beef, buy the leanest cut you can.

Chicken

Free-range chickens are better than conventional chickens that live in tight buildings. Conventional chickens are traditionally fed grains and antibiotics to grow bigger and survive the tough conditions. Additionally, conventionally raised chickens are loaded with chemicals and tend to have more unhealthy fats than organic, free-range, or pasture-raised chicken.

Free-range chickens are allowed to walk around outside and have a diet that combines natural grass and plants with their feed. Organic chickens, the next step up, are free-range and have been raised in a natural environment—no antibiotics allowed. And pasture-raised, the best of all, means that the chickens are not only allowed to roam but eat only what they would in the wild, mostly seeds, weeds, and bugs.

So if you can, buy free-range or pasture-raised eggs and chickens. You'll notice a difference in how they taste—and for eggs, even how they look. Factory-farm egg yolks are usually a light yellow, whereas free-range eggs and pasture-raised eggs are a much deeper yellow from the extra beta-carotene they contain.

Fish

When it comes to fish, wild is better. It's leaner and has more omega-3s as a percentage of total fat than farmed fish. Salmon is a great example: farmed salmon has much more fat than wild salmon. Farmed salmon has omega-3s, but also contains a lot of omega-6s (fats we should limit). Omega-3s and omega-6s both wind up in our cell membranes, and how much we eat of each one determines whether the healthy, anti-inflammatory omega-3s dominate or whether the inflammatory omega-6s dominate. In farmed fish, there are loads of omega-6s that skew the balance; in wild fish, the omega-3s vastly outnumber the omega-6s. So while eating a farmed fish would be better than a grain-fed steak or a factory-farm chicken breast, it's not nearly as healthy as wild fish.

Toxins are one of the main reasons that nutritionists don't advocate eating fish for every meal. If you focus on eating the smaller fish on the food chain such as salmon and haddock rather than the larger ones such as tuna and Chilean sea bass, you'll avoid the problems associated with the toxins in fish, such as mercury. On the Cheat System, I'd love for you to try eating fish once a week. And be sure to take fish oil capsules for an extra dose of omega-3s that will push your weight loss in the right direction.

Pea/Rice Protein

It's a complete protein, has the same amount of branched-chain amino acids as meat, and it's a great shortcut for breakfast. It fills you up and the protein releases slowly. In fact, pea protein releases more slowly than the whey protein in most "energy" shakes, which makes you feel fuller longer.

IS WHEY OR SOY PROTEIN AS GOOD AS PEA/RICE OR PEA/POTATO PROTEIN?

Pea and rice protein, when mixed together, form a complete protein (pea is low in sulfur-containing amino acids while rice is high). Brian Rigby explains, "while whey and soy are also complete proteins, they have a high allergenic nature.

Soy can cause sensitivities and inflammation, and the soy protein isolate used in soy protein powder can also be higher in isoflavones than soy products that have not been processed and concentrated like soy protein isolate has been."

Whey does not contain isoflavones, but can still be a trigger for sensitivities in certain people. Because whey protein is rapidly absorbed, most of it will end up as nitrogen waste in the urine unless you are a serious athlete and just going to or returning from exercise! Pea/rice protein, on the other hand, is digested and absorbed more slowly, causing it to be more satiating for people trying to lose weight and ensuring that the majority of it goes toward maintaining lean body mass, not getting excreted as waste.

Pea/rice protein is highly digestible and readily absorbed. If you are concerned about exercise and protein for recovery, pea/rice protein is as high in the branched-chain amino acids (BCAAs), arginine, and lysine as whey protein, making it equal in terms of muscle recovery, strength training, and fat burning.

And remember . . . if you're having a PEERtrainer Cheat System–approved shake recipe, you earn an entire cheat!

3. Unlimited Eats: The Star of the Show

Eat Your Eats—as much as you want, any time you want. Berries, cucumbers, grapefruit, artichokes, spinach, Swiss chard, asparagus, butternut squash, sweet potato fries, peppers, salsa, kale, mushrooms. There's no need to portion control these foods, because the Eats work on so many different levels for weight loss. If you want to eat an entire package of berries for breakfast, you can! If you wanted to bake sweet potato fries, you can eat as many as you want! The possibilities are endless for delicious Eats that are low in calories, keep you feeling full—and are high in the minerals, vitamins, and phytonutrients that your body needs to be healthy, including antioxidants. These foods are unlimited, unlimited, unlimited—because the Eats are nature's diet pill.

Eating the Eats, and the Cheat System way of eating as a whole, helps you lose weight across the board by making the process of weight loss natural and easy for your body. If you eat three meals a day that contain the protein your body needs to maintain itself, the healthy fats that make you feel satiated, and the Eats that keep you full, reduce your inflammation, and stabilize the physiological responses like cortisol and insulin, at every level the Cheat System makes it easy for your body to lose the excess weight.

UNLIMITED EATS, "GOOD" FAT, "TRADITIONAL" PROTEIN, AND CHEATS ON TOP!

Every time you look at your plate, it's almost all Eats

So you now have a sense of what your plate looks like: unlimited Eats, "good" fat, and a "traditional" protein, and of course, your Cheats on top. Bacon. Or Parm crisps. Or goat cheese. It's all a part of it.

All that's required for the Cheat System to "work" for you, in terms of diet, is that you focus on your Eats and your Free Cheats (more on this later). This equation combines the work of researchers and doctors who have studied successful weight loss and the experiences of real-life people who have successfully lost weight. It's the marriage of what's been clinically proven to work, and what works in the real world.

On the Cheat System, you don't have to count calories for your Eats, you don't have to worry about fiber or fat, and you don't even have to eliminate foods. We have done the hard work for you. All you have to do is Eat your Eats, which is most of your meal, and limit your Cheats. Seems pretty simple, right?

In Chapter 4, we'll go into the entire plan and show you exactly how to eat to lose up to twelve pounds in three weeks. The Cheat System Diet has worked for thousands of PEERtrainer members, and it will work for you. We've mastered the hardest part of losing weight: making a diet doable in the real world, and making it easy for you to follow through on your intentions and goals to get healthy. As *Men's Health* says, "Abs are made in the kitchen," and 75 percent of weight loss is making sure you eat your Eats. In the next chapter, I'll show you what makes up the remaining 25 percent.

CHAPTER 3

Pain Equals Gain

Why You Work Out, Stress Out, and Lose Nothing—And Why Cheating Will "Work Out" for You

If you're not taking care of you, you're not in a position to help anyone else. You can't give what you don't have . . .

—STEVE SIEBOLD

Maybe you think you can't lose weight because you don't think you have the workout "gene" or because you don't have professional help at the gym. You're not like my best friend from high school who used to work out for three hours every day. You're not like your neighbor, who puts on his running shoes and goes out for a run on Saturday mornings. You think these people aren't like you, are never going to be you, and you'll just get by with whatever you can do.

Or maybe you think you know what to do when you work out. You know that you should lift weights twice a week, do cardio three or four days a week, and do interval training. Maybe you're the type of person who competes in triathlons just for fun, or to see how far you can push yourself.

Whether you're the kind of person who does marathons for fun or the kind of person who thinks you would die trying to run a mile, *fitness fusion*, aka the Cheat System Exercise Plan, will not only help you lose weight but will also motivate you to move and help keep you from being sidelined in the future.

Just like the Diet Fusion concept you learned about in the previous chapter, *Fitness Fusion* combines the best of what's out there into a plan that not only works, but is actually doable in real life.

Fitness fusion works because it utilizes the number one secret professional athletes, top coaches, and trainers know: that by working out *at your baseline* (more on this later) **you burn more fat—while avoiding fatigue and preventing injury.**

"BUT I'LL GAIN WEIGHT IF I WORK OUT LESS!"

A lot of people freak out when they learn that the Cheat System Exercise Plan asks them to fight the "no pain, no gain" strategy, because they are worried any reduction in what they are doing will cause them to gain weight.

But in reality, when you do the right kind of exercise, at the right speed and the right intensity for your individual body, each workout you do will be more productive for weight loss—and once you see those results, the stress you feel about working out will also decrease because you'll know that what you're doing works!

THE FOUR PILLARS TO FITNESS FUSION

You don't have to become a gym rat or a marathoner or someone who goes to yoga five times a week in order to make Cheat System fitness plan work for you. In fact, the opposite is true! At PEERtrainer, we've found that combining the four pillars to fitness fusion is all you need to do in order to make a workout *truly* productive.

+ Build your base.
+ Get your body aligned and in balance (to ease pain and prevent injury).
+ Find the movement and fitness you love.
+ Confront your stress.

Build Your Base

Building your base is exactly the opposite of the "no pain, no gain" mantra everyone thinks works. The mantra that says: Thirty minutes on the treadmill is better than twenty; working out at the gym five days a week is better than three. You see it all over any gym in America, from the guy squatting gigantic weights to the girl suffering on the treadmill. Even the "inspirational" signs posted in most gyms promote the idea that in order to exercise "right" you have to in some way burn and churn and huff and puff your way through it.

But the truth is that while you may lose some weight when you work out this way, physiologically you create conditions where all your body wants to do is put that weight back on. The traditional exercise narrative of "no pain, no gain" and "more is better" simply does not help most of us lose weight and keep it off.

Have you ever been at the gym on a treadmill or the elliptical and seen a graph that shows your fat-burning state zone versus the aerobic zone based on your heart rate? When your heart rate goes over a certain number, your body has less oxygen during the workout. But to burn fat, you need oxygen. If you're working out too hard, your body has less oxygen and it starts to burn sugar rather than fat. If you're huffing and puffing and burning it out, you're no *longer* burning fat. You're burning sugar.

Remember cortisol from Chapter 1? It relates to your exercise here. *All exercise raises your cortisol levels.* All of it. So you might be asking, "Well, if this is true, then why am I exercising at all?" But cortisol isn't bad: it's a natural hormone that protects you—when its levels are normal. But when cortisol levels are too high, it keeps the belly fat on.

Our body automatically releases cortisol in order to make sure our brain has fuel. If we're working out at the right intensity, our cortisol does its job and we lose weight. (In fact, a study in the *Journal of Endocrinological Investigation* has shown that low-intensity exercise may actually *lower* cortisol levels—great news!)

But if we're working out too hard or too fast, our body increases the amount of cortisol in our body. Having excess cortisol encourages your body to store those calories, potentially destroying any benefits you've gained from exercise!

That's why it's *so* important to build your base. If you know what your base is, you won't pass the place where your body burns more sugar than fat, and you won't increase the amount of cortisol in your blood and later add fat to your belly. A study published in the *International Journal of Sports Physiology and Performance* backs this up: it showed that high-intensity exercise stimulates a greater increase in cortisol than workouts that are not as intense. Even more important, cortisol also been shown to increase over time the longer you work out, by a study published in the medical journal *Brain Research*.

You can properly work out, raise your cortisol levels, and still be in a fat-burning zone. How?

Let me explain something very briefly here. As Stu Mittleman, the ultramarathoner and athlete who completed a 1,000-mile run in ten days (running 100 miles every single day for ten days straight!), explains, you have two types of energy reserves: you have sugar reserves and you have fat reserves. You need both. Your sugar reserves help you with your fight-and-flight response; they give you that superhuman energy when you're in trouble (like when we had to run from a tiger way back when). But we have virtually limitless amount of fat reserves. It's better to get our energy to exercise from our fat reserves, but what do most people do? They go way over their own individual baseline and they work out as hard as they can. They're accessing all their sugar (fight-or-flight) reserves, rather than their limitless fat reserves.

So now you might be wondering, what about people who can run a seven-minute mile? They're going as fast as they can. And they're skinny as a rail. Here's the catch: it's not about how fast you're going. It's about how fast your body is *ready* to go. We all have a different baseline of physical fitness, where you're working out and burning fat or you're working out and burning sugar. With the PEERtrainer Cheat System fitness plan, we're going to teach you how to get into this fat-burning zone.

Most people cannot do high-intensity exercise properly without first building up their base level of fitness. What do I mean by base level of fitness? Your base level of fitness is where you are comfortable exercising, where you can finish a workout and feel like it was so easy that you could go out and do it again. It feels good; it's pleasurable. Okay, maybe you couldn't do the entire thing again, but you don't want to pass out. You don't have tunnel vision, which means you aren't staring into space like a zombie, without any thoughts at all except wondering how much time you have left. You aren't praying for the workout to be over. There's an ease and flow.

So how can you tell what your base is? You can figure that out by being honest with yourself, trying different kinds of exercise, and answering our Are You Working Out Too Hard, Too Fast? quiz below. If you've been a couch potato for a few years, your base will definitely be lower than someone who goes to the gym four times a week—which is normal and totally okay.

Are You Working Out Too Hard, Too Fast?

Most of the ten questions below are pretty easy to answer even if you haven't worked out in a few days, weeks, or even months—but if you do work out sometime in the next day or two, it can be useful to revisit this questionnaire afterward to see how many questions really pertain to you. (Most people identify with a few initially, and then realize after working out that they identify with even more.)

1. During a workout, do you become red-faced or are huffing and puffing and find it hard to breathe?

2. Are you ravenous after a workout? Do you want to eat a Coke or cheeseburger or a huge bowl of pasta afterward? Or do you just feel like, "Oh, I could eat a salad"?

3. Do you have to force yourself to finish what you set out to do, no matter what? And if you do quit early, do you beat yourself up about it for the rest of the day, or think something like "I have to make that up"?

4. Do you have blinders on? Do you have trouble noticing the people, the landscape, and/or the scenery around you while working out? Can you look around while you're working out, or do you have to look straight ahead the entire time in order

to make it through? Is your mind a blank when you work out—almost virtually no thoughts?

5. Is music necessary for you to even think of finishing your workout? Could you work out without having headphones on or a television blaring in front of you?

6. Do you feel constrained by time? (Do you always think something like "How do I find an hour to do this?" when you are trying to get a workout in?)

7. Are you getting injured? Injury can mean anything from a slight strain that causes you to skip a workout or two to a muscle tear or pain that sidelines you for months.

8. Are you getting sick more than once every six to eight weeks?

9. How much do you have to motivate yourself to go work out? Do you have to push yourself or convince yourself to go every single time?

10. Do you have an unreasonable amount of fat around your abdomen?

If you answered yes to or identified with more than four questions, you are working out far beyond your base—either trying to do too much or moving too fast, both of which are completely counterproductive to burning fat while you work out and may set you up for injury.

I know some of you will say that hard workouts are your only stress reliever. I get it—and if you're at the weight you want to be at, fine. But overexercising has a massive effect on your weight—and actually works as a stressor, not as a way to de-stress. Doing a hard, long workout over your baseline that causes your body more stress than it relieves is like putting a Band-Aid on a gaping wound—helpful, but definitely not effective in the long run.

Finding Your Base—and Building It

It's pretty simple to find your base: try different forms of exercise, at different speeds. When you can answer no to at least seven of the questions above, you've found a workout that matches your base.

Once you've found where your base level is, you can build it simply by adding small challenges to your workout. If you've been inactive and you're starting out by simply walking, adding a short minute-long jog at the end of your walk is a great way to build your base. That minute is what is commonly called sprinting. If you've been going to the gym consistently, you could build your base by attending a different class or doing a workout outside like cycling or walking in a park. During your workout, you should be in the fat-burning state (what we described above) at least 85 percent of the time. Fifteen percent of the time, you can be in that huff-and-puff sugar-burning state where you're moving faster. However, a quick indicator that you're in good heart health, according to Dr. Steven Masley, is if you're able to run up a hill. So, if you're interested in just getting and staying fit, being able to run up a hill is a great goal.

And once you know what your base is, you can build upon what you're able to do.

THE BEST EXERCISE EVER!

Whether you've been working out or not, walking is the perfect example of a "slow workout" that will maximize fat burning while building your base. As you continue to walk, your fitness will improve allowing you to walk longer or faster without stressing your body.

If you're already working out or following a training program you like, walking is perfect for cross-training. And if you're just starting out, it's a great way to build your base before exploring more high-intensity forms of exercise.

So What Is the Cheat System Fat-Burning Workout?

If you suspect that you've been working out too hard or too fast, the first change you should make to your workouts is to simply *slow down*. When you slow it down and build your base over time, you teach your body how to access the fat-burning side. Not only do you stop craving sugar and junk food after working out, but you also decrease your body's overall stress and cortisol levels—helping you to lose weight.

If you've been working out, you can continue to do your current workouts on the Cheat System. But you must be able to answer no to at least seven questions in that quiz to know you're in the fat-burning zone.

If you haven't worked out in a long time or you suspect you've been burning sugar, not fat, because you often have injuries (such as knee, back, and/or shoulder pain) or you're completely not motivated to do anything, I want you to **walk twenty minutes every other day.** You don't have to do it all at one time. It can be ten minutes here, ten minutes there. You can take the stairs instead of the elevator. I want you to start feeling good about movement again on the Cheat System. The eight-minute mile may come later or you may never want to pursue that. That's okay. Don't beat yourself up for not liking a certain sport. Later in the chapter, we teach you how to love working out by finding the sport you love. But for the next three weeks, I want you to just commit to twenty minutes of walking every other day.

Get Your Body Aligned and Balanced (to Ease Pain and Prevent Injury)

Far too often, I'll be sitting with people and someone will say, "I slipped and fell earlier this week. I hurt my knee and I can barely walk, even though I'm on painkillers and am keeping my knee elevated. Should I go to the MRI now or later? I know I won't be able to work out for three months."

Or a PEERtrainer member will post something like this on one of our forums: "Walking is too hard for me. I'm in so much pain; I'm trying to keep a positive attitude, but I can't think of anything other than that I'm in pain and can't do anything about it."

Every time I have one of these conversations, it breaks my heart because I've learned that chronic pain is often the body's way of telling us it's out of balance—and getting out of pain often isn't another painkiller or surgery or MRI. It's getting your body aligned and back in balance.

HOW DO WE KNOW WHEN WE'RE OUT OF BALANCE?

As we get out of balance, we avoid things. We might avoid climbing ladders, taking the stairs, craning our neck to see something, checking our mirrors in our car, avoiding hills when we're outside walking, avoiding anything new or challenging that we are not sure of physically. Another indicator, as told to me by Pete Egoscue, one of the world's leading experts at stopping chronic pain, is the direction your feet point. Stand up. If your feet point at ten and two, or even nine and three, this is an indication that your movement is inefficient and your body might not be in alignment.

At PEERtrainer, many of our members are skeptical that injuries could be related to the body's alignment and balance and can be healed without going to the doctor and getting painkillers.

But I'm here to tell you—from experience—that it's possible to heal yourself and recover from injury or pain without endless trips to a physical therapist or a doctor and/or living on painkillers. And it's not just me. Athletes like Jack Nicklaus, Eli Manning, and even Bethany Hamilton, the surfer who lost her arm, have used these same methods to eliminate their daily pain.

I experienced pain and injury—and recovered—twice. The first time happened when I was twenty-five years old and was reasonably fit. I windsurfed. I would run in Central Park most days of the week. One day I bent down to pull something out of a dresser and was completely debilitated.

Everyone told me to get a back brace and to do physical therapy, so I did. My doctor said I should never run again and that I would experience back pain every day for the rest of my life. I came home from work and spent every night just lying on my couch. My workouts were reduced to a half hour on the recumbent bike and I was miserable.

After eight months of living this way, one afternoon I came home and got really mad. I had wanted and expected to live a really active life well into my nineties, maybe even over a hundred—my grandmother was in her eighties and was still working out at Gold's Gym! So I knew you could be older and still be very active. As I lay down on the sofa, with my back brace on, all I could think was "I can't live like this."

I heard about Dr. John Sarno on the radio. I was desperate for anything that could help me and quickly bought the book. After doing Dr. Sarno's exercises from his book *Healing Back Pain*, I was about 85 percent healed—a huge jump from the 10 percent I had recovered from physical therapy.

What Dr. Sarno (who is the bestselling author of numerous books, professor of Rehabilitation Medicine at the New York University School of Medicine, and an attending physician at New York University Medical Center) says is that a lot of pain—particularly in the knees, neck, shoulders, and back—is caused by our emotions, not by any structural injuries that can be seen by an MRI or helped by medical interventions or physical therapy.

In an interview we did with Dr. Sarno for PEERtrainer, he explained that many people have anger at an unconscious level. Our brain wants to distract itself from the unconscious anger but also to draw our conscious attention to it, so it funnels signals to the nerves in our muscles, which cause the pain. This can cause muscle pain, headaches, allergic reactions, and gastrointestinal ailments.

Most of us focus on medical interventions and see doctors in hope of relieving our pain, but that doesn't help if the pain is caused by psychological issues, which Dr. Sarno contends happens with most people most of the time. So how can you figure out whether your pain is caused by emotional stress or by an actual, structural injury that needs intervention?

First, ignore the pain for a few days. This may sound like exactly what you don't want to do, but you need to ignore the pain and treat what could be the underlying symptom: the stress and anger in your life. Let's face it: our culture isn't supportive of anger even when it's completely justified. A lot of people don't feel like they have the right to feel angry, but if you give yourself permission to experience and express that anger, the physical pain caused by your psychological stress will dissipate.

Acknowledge your feelings (I'm angry about this) and that it's okay to feel that way (I'm upset that this happened) without minimizing how you feel. So many of us minimize how we feel, push it down inside, or simply don't get anger *out*. Often expressing anger requires you to stop saying what you're always told to say.

Sometimes we've repressed so many of our feelings that we don't even know what we're mad about. When can you tell this is happening? When you get emotional in an irrational way. If you lose it with your husband when he doesn't do something very small you asked him to, or when you break down watching a television show. In those moments, you can usually begin to figure out "What am I really mad about?"

Once you are able to acknowledge that the mind has a lot to do with physical pain, you should see a gradual decline of your pain over the span of a few weeks, like I did. A peer-reviewed study showed that more than half of the patients who used Dr. Sarno's techniques to treat chronic back pain felt noticeable relief and/or full recovery from their previous symptoms.

DISCLAIMER: PLEASE USE COMMON SENSE

You always could have a real injury and need to see a doctor. I pursued these methods after a doctor could not see anything acutely wrong.

That being said, Dr. Sarno is just one piece of the pain puzzle. I wasn't settling for 85 percent. I wanted to be out of pain. A friend of mine worked with Tony Robbins, and he told me he learned how to eliminate pain from a good friend of his, Pete Egoscue.

Pete Egoscue is a really special human being. He is a military veteran wounded in Vietnam who figured out how to cure his own war injury. He's the one who Jack Nicklaus credits for his having the longest career of any professional golfer. Egoscue believes that we should all, no matter what our age, be as agile as little kids. That's because little kids move naturally and use all of their muscles, both the primary and the complementary muscles constantly. But adults tend to move in the same way every day and rely only on their primary muscles (think of the elliptical at the gym or just sitting at your computer), which allows our complementary muscles to atrophy. You'll see kids roll down hills, climb under tables, and move in a lot of different ways daily. Even if you're fit, you're most likely using the same kind of complementary muscles over and over again, so the muscles you don't use may be atrophied.

When I was twenty-five, I went to one of Egoscue's clinics and, with his methods, was able to completely heal my back. Sarno helped me get to 85 percent, and after Egoscue I was 100 percent back. I could in-line skate again. I could run and ski. I haven't looked at another recumbent bike since.

Egoscue works with some of the most famous athletes in the world, and his methods are popular with a lot of people like me whose lives have been changed by his clinics. I promise you, if you're in any kind of pain at all, from chronic to just a nagging ache in your back, the exercises we share below will help. When you begin to do the Cheat System exercises, you will feel relief from your pain. Even if you're thinking "it won't work for me," think about this: you don't have anything to lose from trying the exercises, but you do have something to lose from living in pain.

WHY CHIROPRACTORS FEEL *SOOO* GOOD

The reason we feel good after going to a chiropractor is because a chiropractor forces your back into perfect alignment. But that doesn't fix the atrophied muscles you have in complementary muscles you're not using. If you don't strengthen those muscles, you will soon be out of alignment and you won't feel better until you go back to the chiropractor again. But the menu of exercises we are sharing from Pete Egoscue focus on all those complementary muscles and gradually put you back in alignment again. A lot have small, odd movements that make you feel good—so that you can hike up a hill, fall down on a rock, and not injure yourself for life—and you'll save some money at the chiropractor.

THE EGOSCUE THREE-WEEK PLAN

Brian Bradley and the staff at Egoscue in San Diego have put together an exclusive plan for people following the Cheat System. It's a three-week plan designed to get you aligned properly so you can pursue whatever physical activity you want and have physical confidence.

It's important to realize that when you work out without stretching or flexibility exercises like those in the Egoscue plan, you end up building your primary muscles without building any secondary muscles—which results in your body not being in balance and sometimes injured. Building primary muscles only is like building a roof with rafters, but skipping the shingles. The rain will come in. So to protect your entire body from the rain (injuries), I'd like for you to do four stretches that work on your body's alignment. I'd like you to do them every other day.

What these stretches do is build the ancillary and secondary muscles that support you during activity. The only way to be truly fit and aligned (which naturally lowers cortisol) is to exercise and move these muscles. The alignment exercises balance out the use of our primary muscles (while we exercise) by working the complementary muscles as well—this helps to minimize pain and protect against injury throughout your body. You don't need any special equipment to do these stretches, and the whole routine should take under ten minutes. This is a huge and easy component of why the Cheat System Exercise Plan works.

THE EGOSCUE THREE-WEEK PLAN DESIGNED FOR THE CHEAT SYSTEM

There are twelve stretches in this menu, created especially for readers of this book. Do the exercises in this plan according to this schedule:

- Week One: Do exercises 1 to 4 every other day (every day if you can—it's only ten minutes!)
- Week Two: Do exercises 5 to 8 every other day (every day if you can—it's only ten minutes!)
- Week Three: Do exercises 9 to 12 every other day (every day if you can—it's only ten minutes!)

WEEK ONE

1. Standing Arm Circles

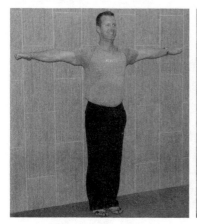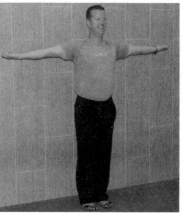

Two sets of 40 repetitions each.

Stand with your feet pointed straight and hip-width apart.

Place your fingertips into the palm of each hand and point your thumbs straight out (this hand position is important for the exercise to be done correctly).

Pull your shoulders back by squeezing your shoulder blades together, then bring your arms out straight from your sides up to shoulder level.

With palms facing down and your thumbs pointing straight forward, rotate your hands up and forward in approximately six-inch circles. Do twenty reps.

Then reverse direction: palms should face up, with thumbs pointed straight backward. Rotate your hands up and backward. Do twenty reps.

2. Standing Elbow Curls

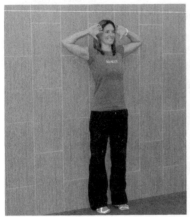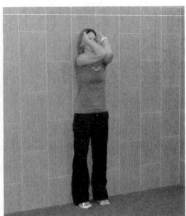

One set of 25 repetitions.

Stand at a wall with your heels, hips, upper back, and head against the wall. Your feet should be pointed straight and hip-width apart.

Place your knuckles against your temples with your thumbs pointing down toward your shoulders (your fingertips should be touching your palm as they were on the last exercise).

Open and pull back your elbows so that they are against the wall, then close your elbows together in front of your face. (Be sure that your elbows stay at shoulder level—don't let them drop down!)

Repeat for twenty-five reps.

3. Airbench

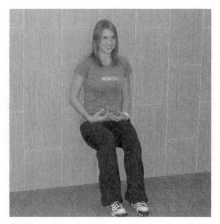

Hold this stretch for two minutes.

Stand with your back against a wall with feet and knees hip-width apart and feet pointed straight.

Walk your feet away from the wall while sliding your body down at the same time. You will be "seated" in an invisible chair; your knees should be bent at about 105 degrees (a little wider than a right angle). Your hips should be just slightly higher than your knees and your ankles slightly ahead of your knees. Your lower back should be completely against the wall. Your arms can hang down or be placed gently in your lap.

Keep your weight on your heels.

Be sure to do this exercise in athletic shoes or on a yoga mat. Don't try it in socks or bare feet—you might slip!

4. Assisted Runners Stretch

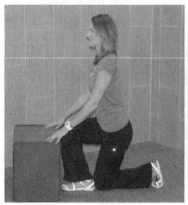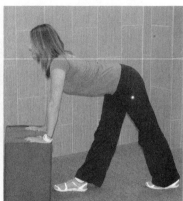

Hold this stretch for one minute.

Kneel down in front of a chair or table that you can use to stabilize and support your body.

Place the back of your right heel on the front of your left knee. Be sure that you are up on the toes of your left foot, with the bottom of your foot pointing behind you. Keep your right foot, your left knee, and your left foot in line with each other.

Keeping your hands on the chair, stand up and begin bending over while rolling your hips back, which will make an arch in your lower back. The heel of your left foot should be on the ground.

Tighten your thighs (quads) while relaxing your upper body. Keep your weight on the inside of each foot, and keep your lower back arched.

Hold for one minute; switch sides and repeat.

WEEK TWO

5. Cats and Dogs

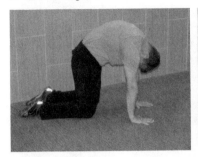 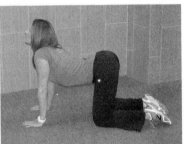

One set of ten repetitions.

Start on your hands and knees. Be sure that your hips are directly above your knees, and that your shoulders are directly above your hands. Your fingers should be pointed forward.

Move into *cat* by pulling your hips under, pulling your head under, and pushing your upper back to the ceiling to round your back. Exhale.

Then move into *dog* by rolling your hips forward, putting an arch in your back, and collapsing your shoulder blades together. Look up. Inhale.

Move from cat to dog ten times for the full set.

6. Downward Dog

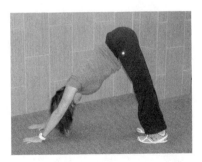

Hold this exercise for one minute.

Start on your hands and knees. Your hands should be directly below your shoulders; your knees should be in line with your hips.

Pull your toes under to grip the floor, and pull your knees off the floor into the pike position.

Your knees should be straight. The goal is to pull your upper body through your arms toward the floor. Though your heels do not need to touch the floor, this is the intended position (and can be a goal to work toward).

Concentrate on trying to roll your hips forward to place an arch in your lower back, tighten your thighs, and hold for 1 minute.

7. Hip Lift

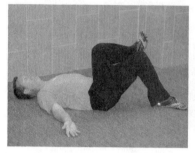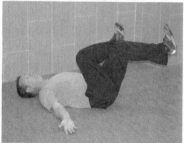

Hold for one minute on each side of your body.

Lie on your back with your feet on the floor. Cross one ankle/foot just above the opposite knee, and place it just above the knee on your leg.

Lift the foot that is still on the floor up until your calf is parallel to the ground, and your knee is bent at a ninety-degree angle. Relax your shoulders and put your arms out to your side, palms facing up.

As you pull the knee with your ankle on it toward you, press the other knee away. Hold for one minute, then switch sides and repeat.

8. Hip Crossover Stretch

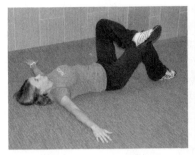 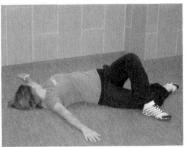

Hold this stretch for one minute on each side of your body.

Lie on your back with both knees bent and your feet flat on the floor, pointed ahead. Place your arms out to the side at shoulder level, with your palms facing down, flat on the floor.

Cross your left ankle over your right knee and rotate the ankle/knee junction down toward the floor. Your left foot should now be flat on the floor, along with the outside of your right leg.

Look in the opposite direction and relax your shoulders. Press the left knee away from your body using your left hip muscles.

Hold for one minute, then switch sides and repeat.

WEEK THREE

9. One-Arm Bridge

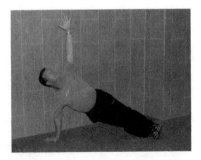

Hold for one minute on each side of the body.

Lie on your side with the hand that is under your body on the floor slightly ahead of your shoulder.

Stack your feet so the outside of one foot is on the floor and the other foot is stacked on top of it. (You can rest your feet against a wall if you need to.)

Prop yourself up onto one hand so your arm is fully extended. When your arm is extended, your hand will be in front of your shoulder.

Raise your other arm to the ceiling and look up. Keep your hip and pelvis in line; as you get tired, try not to let them drop toward the floor.

Hold for one minute, then switch sides and repeat.

10. Static Back

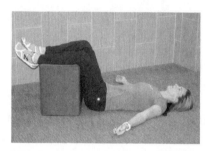

Hold for five minutes.

Lie on your back with your legs up over a block or a chair.

Place your arms out to your sides about forty-five degrees away from your body with your palms facing up.

Relax your upper back, and notice if your lower back flattens to the floor evenly from left to right. Hold for five minutes.

11. Static Back Pull-Overs

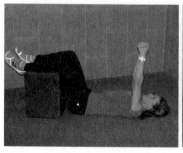 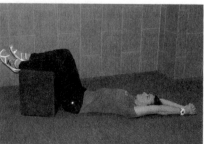

Three sets of ten repetitions each.

Lie on your back with your legs up over a block or a chair so that your legs are bent at a right angle. Relax your legs, lower back, and stomach.

Reach your arms straight above your chest, elbows locked, and hands clasped together.

Lower your hands down to the floor above your head. Do not contract your abdominal muscles; keep your stomach and lower back relaxed. Do not let your arms bend at the elbow. If you are not able to lower your hands all the way to the floor behind you, go only as low as you are able to with straight arms. Raise your arms back to starting position. Do ten reps in each set.

12. Upper Spinal Floor Twist

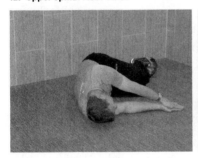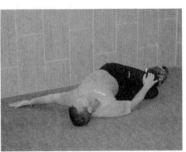

Hold for one minute on each side.

Lie on your side in the fetal position, with your arms held straight out from your shoulders in front of you.

Stack your knees directly atop one another, where they should remain throughout the exercise.

Open your top arm, lifting it up and over your body to the other side, letting it rest on the floor (or as close to the floor as you're able). Your shoulders and torso will follow; however, don't move your lower body from the previous position. Feel free to use your bottom hand to hold your knees together.

Move your head to look in the same direction as your top arm. Breathe deeply and evenly; allow your body to open up.

Hold for one minute and repeat on the other side.

This is a basic introduction to the Egoscue stretches. You can find more in Dr. Egoscue's book, *Pain Free*, or visit an Egoscue clinic to create your own personalized menu.

Find the Movement and Fitness You Love

If you really embrace the ideas from the first two fitness pillars, this third step will probably come easily. You will find that you *want* to move more, and you will be open to the possibility that exercise doesn't have to be boring, that it can be fun.

When you enjoy the feeling of exercise, you are motivated for life. When you start doing a workout that you like, you may begin to realize why some people claim to love exercise. And that's because those people know about *flow*.

Flow: How to Make Exercise Fun

Although athletes call flow different things—being in the zone and runner's high—flow is when your body and mind come together to make exercise engaging, fulfilling, and entertaining. When you work out at your physical base level, like you will on the Cheat System exercise plan, it will be easier to experience flow.

Being in a flow state is an easy way to become even more physically fit than you ever thought possible, because it makes exercise doable both physically and mentally. And though you'll notice that flow states require you to slow down at first, the more flow workouts you do the faster you will get without injury and without wanting to quit.

It's easiest to experience flow when you are doing an activity that you love. If you aren't enjoying your workout routine now, think of what you liked doing when you were younger. For example, growing up, I danced almost every day—tap, jazz, ballet—but at some point, I just gave it up. So I bought the video game Dance Party. I can do it by myself, or suggest it when people come over. I bought Wii Tennis for the same reason. I don't need a court or a partner or good weather, just the Wii. And when I'm doing those things, I'm moving, which is what really matters.

Jonathan Fields, a partner at PEERtrainer who specializes in and has written books about flow, says that being in flow requires absorption and mental focus while still having fun. Most mainstream fitness routines prevent flow by being rote activities that are really boring—a treadmill is a great example. The reason treadmills have televisions that most people plug into and tune out on is because the exercise is so boring!

In contrast, running outside—or better yet, running on a trail—requires your full attention and engages you. You have to concentrate on where you're running or else you'll run into a tree or stumble on a rock and fall. Because you're outside, your surroundings change, keeping you interested in what's happening around you. That mental engagement is rewarding and satisfying—which encourages you to keep going, to finish the workout, and especially to come back for more another day.

By its very nature, flow is a bit mystifying until it happens to you. But there are eight requirements to flow, which Jonathan Fields, the founder of the Good Life Project, first explained to me (which I've included below). These eight stages have to happen in combination with each other (nearly simultaneously) in order for you to enter a flow state. It's important to note, though, that flow isn't just for exercise: it can happen at work, when you're in conversation with a good friend, when you're playing a musical instrument or knitting a scarf or practicing a craft or writing a story, or doing anything that requires both creativity and focus.

THE EIGHT STAGES OF FLOW

1. Clear Goals

You know what you want to achieve and what the rules of the activity are, even if you set those boundaries for yourself. For example, a tennis player knows the rules of the game and wants to beat his or her opponent; if you're walking, you could have set a goal of being able to walk faster than before, or simply to walk for a certain length of time.

2. High Concentration

You're focused solely on what you're doing, not what else you have to do during the day or what has been weighing on your mind prior to the activity. You're intensely focused on what you're doing and how it is making your body feel.

3. It's Hard But Not Tough

There's a balance between the activity requiring the skills you already have and being challenging at the same time. So if you are playing tennis you could have a worthy opponent who is slightly better than you; if you're walking, you're keeping a slightly faster pace than normal, but can still breathe and finish your walk in fat-burning mode.

4. You're In Control

You feel secure and relaxed psychologically while doing the activity. You're not worried about what you look like, what obstacles may be in your path, or what the other people around you think about you or what you're doing.

5. It Feels Effortless

Though the activity may look strenuous to someone else, it doesn't cause any strain to you. And honestly, you realize that you don't need to think about what you're doing all that much while doing it.

6. No Perception of Time

You feel like you could go on forever, or that the amount of time you've spent exercising feels like half of what is showing on your watch or smartphone.

7. A Feeling of Unity

There is no mental room for worry, fear, distraction, or rumination. You feel at peace with your performance, or if participating with others in a group activity, how your team is performing as a whole. You feel deeply connected to what you're doing, like your performance and yourself are one and the same.

8. Immediately Gratifying

When you're finished with the activity, you feel like you could go out and do it again—or want to, just because you want to replicate the feeling you had while you were doing the exercise. This can also happen while you are doing the activity—creating the feeling that you never want to stop.

Each stage of flow can happen independently of the others, so if you decide to try a new exercise, try to be conscious of how you are feeling.

If you lose perception of time, or find yourself feeling super pumped up and wanting to do that activity again when you finish your workout, those are great indicators that whatever activity you're doing could induce a flow state should you keep doing it.

While it doesn't matter what kind of exercise or activity you are doing when you are able to get into flow, being in a flow state helps your body supercharge fat burning (and lower cortisol) because you're moving at the right pace and you are totally relaxed. If you've never been in flow state before, start with a mental or physical activity that is appealing and easy for you to do. It can be drawing. It can be tennis. Something that makes you feel great.

Walking can often induce flow states and provide you with the mental space you need to clear clutter that's been causing stress. As a general rule, classes are more inclined to create flow states than the rote workout equipment at the gym. Any activity you think that you "should" do but worry that you might get hurt doing or really dislike is an activity that is the opposite of flow. You are in flow when you feel great and you're doing well.

Zumba, yoga, team sports, and even cardio body-sculpting classes can induce group flow states—where everyone in the room is in flow— which have even more powerful effects on weight loss.

Confront Your Stress

If you learn nothing else from this chapter, I want you to realize that you're probably working out much harder than you think you are. You also work out more often than you think, too—because not only is the time you spend actually exercising a workout, but every time you *stress* out is a workout, too!

Your Stress Is a Workout (and Your Workout Is Stress)

A lot of the "workouts" we do on a daily basis don't happen at a gym. A workout is happening when you have a fight with your mom on the phone, and end up pacing back and forth as you argue with her.

The second you focus on something that's out of your control, whether it's the fact that yoga class you like is now scheduled at the same time as pickup for your daughter's school, or that you can't afford the gym membership that all of your colleagues have, I want you to think of that thought process as a workout that's *preventing* you from losing weight. Focusing on things that you can't control sabotages good decision-making and prevents you from losing weight. Period. That ruminating supports the decision to get the large pizza instead of a salad, and the cortisol it produces adds fat to your belly.

Stress holds you back from losing weight just as much, if not more, than sitting on your couch would. The moment you feel stressed, your body responds the same way as it would if you were starting a stressful workout: it releases cortisol.

Five Miles or Five Minutes

Let's say you were super-motivated one morning and went out for a five-mile run. Your hormones would change as you exercised—especially cortisol, as you already know—but you would also experience the positive effects of a physical workout like better cardiovascular fitness, improved insulin sensitivity, an increase in your lean body mass (muscle), and of course a decrease in fat (as long as you're fat burning).

Now let's pretend that instead of going for a run, you looked at Facebook, saw that your ex is getting married, and proceeded to totally stress out about it for five minutes. Your body would react to this stress in the same way it would have reacted to the exercise, but experience none of the physical benefits of the five-mile run. Instead, it would only receive the negative effects of your hormones at work, including increased belly fat.

Your brain and your body simply can't tell the difference between physiological stress caused by physical activity (the five-mile run) and mental stress (the ex-boyfriend getting married). Your body reacts to both situations, physiologically, the same way: it increases cortisol, which starts breaking down your muscle in order to make new glucose (sugar), and it signals to the body that it needs to preserve all of its blood sugar for the brain. Unlike during exercise where your blood sugar might actually be low because of an actual demand for energy, when you are psychologically stressed, your body doesn't need all that extra blood sugar and so stores it as fat, usually into your belly (cortisol's favorite place to deposit fat cells). Think of extreme physiological stress as adding gas to the tank of your car but never starting it!

Stress within our body, whether it's physical or mental, is the worst workout you can do when trying to lose weight. It doesn't matter whether you run five miles at a pace that is way above your physical baseline or ruminate for five minutes because it has the same negative effect. However, I have to say that I see more people putting undue stress on themselves by giving away their power than anything else.

We can give away our power by putting ourselves down in front of others ("I can't eat that cupcake today—you should have seen what a fatty I was last night!"), by saying yes to something when we want to say no or otherwise trying to please people at our own expense. Either way, we decrease the amount of personal power we have to make positive changes for ourselves in our lives.

When you don't stand up for yourself, your dreams and goals, or what you really want and deserve, you give away your power and essentially take a step back from achieving what you really want and becoming who you really want to be. And, from a weight-loss perspective, all that ruminating will hold you back from what your body needs, physiologically, to shed fat.

So, a great piece of advice that I want you to keep in mind while you're on the Cheat System is from personal development coach Joshua Wayne: **"What other people think of me is none of my business."** It's the truth! You can't control what people think of you, so why bother wondering about it? It only holds you back.

The more you concentrate on what you *can* control—and the less mind space you give things that you can't—the more you will feel like you can succeed on Cheat System. You can't help that the magical yoga class is not at the right time for you. But you can control what you put in your mouth and how much you move throughout the day.

I am no stranger to massive stress. As an entrepreneur, and as a wife, daughter, and mother, I encounter a million stresses each and every day. But I've learned that how your body handles stress is directly related to how you react to it, and the way you're reacting to it now is probably keeping that weight on your belly. At some point you have to make a choice and stop ruminating about things that aren't within your control.

At some point you have to acknowledge the damage stress is doing to your body and your goals. You have to say to yourself, "I'm either going to keep stressing out and keep this weight on" or "I'm going to react differently" and learn how to change the way you react.

Tips and Tricks

It's really hard to stop stressing out, but you have to do it to lose the weight. It's not a nice to have, it's a *must*, and it's a critical component of the Cheat System. What works for me? My first trick: "What other people think of me is none of my business." That works when I think someone may be critical of something I'm doing, or when someone actually says something critical to my face.

The second trick I use when I start to freak out is that I ask myself, "Is there anything I can control here?" Most of the time there isn't, and once you realize that, it instantly defuses the situation.

The third trick is a relaxation exercise I learned from sleep experts Mitchell and Olga Stevko. Sit down, take a deep breath, and focus on a color that relaxes you. Put whatever stresses you out in the middle of that color, whether it's a friend or a family member or a task or whatever. Give it an image in your mind and then make it smaller and smaller. You can even "shoot" it with a gun or a cannon if you like. As the stressor disappears, replace it with an image or an idea that makes you happy—and make that image bigger and bigger. This might sound woo-woo, but I find that it's the easiest way to stop stress in its tracks.

What all three of these tricks do is allow for you to control your reaction over an external force or person or situation that you can't control. And that switches the channel for your brain—there's nothing for it to fix. You can also treat things that stress you out or experiences that are negative the same way you treat television shows you don't like: turn it off, change the channel. You can literally change the channel in your mind by thinking of something else.

When I start thinking about things I can't control, I joke to my husband and my friends that the monkeys in my brain are swinging around wildly. I say, "Uh-oh, the monkeys are gathering for the big bash." It allows me to see that the thoughts are out of control—and picturing them as crazy monkeys helps diminish the power of what I was ruminating over.

These are just a few solutions, but I promise that the more open you are to new suggestions that can help you solve problems, overcome obstacles to weight loss, and relieve stress, the more likely your pounds will drop off. It's like everything else in the book: if your solutions were working for you, you wouldn't be reading this book. So don't be afraid to try one of these exercises, or any other stress-reduction techniques you read about in magazines or whatever. Find what works for you and use it—no matter how ridiculous it may seem to other people. Because the better you are able to manage your stress, the better you'll be able to keep the pounds off.

Change Your Mind, Change Your Weight

When you stop beating yourself up, you take yourself off the mental treadmill—and you decrease your stress and the hormones stress triggers. Not worrying incessantly when you skip a workout about whether you'll gain weight, or about what your ex-boyfriend is doing or someone is saying about you, all helps your body maintain the weight it is rather than send your cortisol skyrocketing and make your belly bigger.

It's actually totally fine to miss a workout every once in a while. It's not the end of the world, and you're certainly not a failure. Your weight loss goals will not be diminished by not going for a walk one day or by skipping a Zumba class that doesn't fit into your schedule. When you decide to de-stress your life and don't worry about how you're working out as much as you once did, you will lose more weight.

Our tendency is to be self-deprecating and to put ourselves down for all the things we can't do or aren't able to do. But at PEERtrainer, we try to shift that focus and take you away from negativity toward yourself and more toward positivity. When you think about exercise, concentrate on your base: What can you do? What do you like to do? And when can you do it?

By focusing on that, instead of churning and burning on some machine for an arbitrary amount of time an arbitrary number of days each week, you'll be able to not only enjoy the exercise you're doing but also see the results on your body. It's much more powerful to concentrate on how great you are. Sure, you should understand the negative—about yourself, about exercise, about life—but embracing all the awesome things about you and understanding that there's a balance is the key to chilling out and allowing the Cheat System program as a whole to work for you.

And one final note: being stressed out and ruminating makes it really hard to lose weight, because it could be the biggest reason you might not be sleeping.

A Magic Pill: Sleep

Sleep may be the most important single thing you can do to easily lose weight. Some experts even believe that getting enough sleep nightly is even more important than diet and exercise for health and longevity. A study has shown that people eat 35 percent more when sleep deprived than when they are fully rested. A lack of sleep could be a significant reason why you feel "hungry all day" —because your cortisol is raised when you don't get enough rest.

The most important step you can take right now to establish healthy sleep patterns is to know what your "sleep number" is. How many hours per night do you need to be rested and energized during the day? According to the Stanford Sleep Center, it's between seven and nine hours a night. Your number is probably the amount of sleep you are sleeping each night by the end of a week of vacation. Once you know your sleep number, try this: set your alarm for the same time every day, *including weekends*, that gives you that amount of time to sleep. So, for instance, if you need eight hours of sleep and you have to get up by 7 A.M. for work, you should be in bed at 11 P.M. and set your alarm for 7 A.M. Remember, if you're not sleeping, you're snacking all day.

The most common issue that people face with sleep is the inability to stop racing thoughts while lying in bed, and calming the mind. I call this "calming my monkeys." I know everything is okay when I have a visual of the monkeys no longer partying. They're sitting and watching TV. That relaxation exercise is one of the greatest tools I have. If I'm still awake after that, I try not to get mad because I know the monkeys have to do a workout before I'll be able to sleep.

Also, a side note, please don't eat within at least two to three hours before going to bed. Set your alarm for going to bed, just like you set your alarm to wake up. Don't go to bed with the TV. Read instead.

WHY CHEATING AND EXERCISING WORKS

The most counterintuitive part of the Cheat System program is our exercise plan. You'll be working out at a slower pace, but your results—in terms of weight loss and overall health—will be better because your workouts will burn fat while reducing stress and cortisol. You'll be using all the principles of Fitness Fusion in combination to get the best results you've ever gotten from working out.

But you won't have to muster every bit of your discipline to work out. It won't be a stressful event. And if you don't have time to do your full workout on a particular day, it's okay to cut the time or skip the workout entirely. Yes, you can "cheat" on working out just like you "cheat" on your diet—and you will still lose weight.

Remember: in order to make the Cheat System Exercise Plan work for you in the best possible way, you need to *build your base* (so you don't accidentally do too much, too fast) and *exercise at the right intensity* so you don't overwhelm your body with cortisol.

"I'VE HEARD THAT SPRINTING IS THE BEST WAY TO LOSE WEIGHT. IS THAT TRUE?"

Sort of. Sprinting can be a great way to burn fat as long as you've actually built your base to sprint. Without building a base, you'll find it challenging to exercise as hard as "high-intensity" demands in order to achieve benefits—which can stress your body out, causing cortisol to rise.

In order to determine whether you can get the benefits of sprinting—or any workout with high-intensity intervals—make sure you can answer no to all of the questions on page 62. If you can say no to all those questions while you're doing the high-intensity interval, you're gaining all the benefits from sprinting. But if you're not, you should slow down until you build your base.

High-intensity exercise like sprints can also be a great fat burner, but build your base first and then make sure you do the exercises correctly.

The Truth About Muscles

A lot of people (especially women) focus on cardiovascular workouts and weight-bearing strength training (Pilates, yoga, etc.) instead of traditional weight-lifting workouts. But the truth is that combining strength training with cardiovascular workouts will not only encourage your body to lose weight but also will make you look better in clothes and increase your overall fitness.

Doing a weights workout once or twice a week helps your body grow its lean muscle mass, which is good because lean muscle mass is "expensive" for your body to maintain. Having it consumes a lot of energy.

When your body has more lean muscle mass, it has a faster metabolism and burns more calories (even at rest) than if it had less because it's sucking more gasoline from your engine and doing it faster. Not to mention that lean muscle mass makes you look thin without looking skinny. In fact, most of the people you think are "naturally thin" probably look that way because they have healthy amounts of lean muscle mass.

You can develop lean muscle mass by lifting weights or doing weight-bearing exercises like yoga or Pilates. Strength-training is actually one of the best fat-burning workouts available, because it increases metabolism so much after you're done working out. During the exercise itself, you're primarily burning sugar calories, but afterward, you will burn hundreds of extra fat calories that you simply wouldn't burn if you hadn't done a strength-training exercise.

It's worth noting, though, that most people benefit from lifting lighter weights because research shows that doing more repetitions with a lighter weight ultimately burns more calories than lifting heavier weights fewer times.

And last but not least, if you're worried that lifting weights will make you look like a bodybuilder, I can tell you from experience that it won't happen. Besides, if you start to notice that you're becoming too toned for your personal taste, all you have to do is skip a couple weight workouts and your body will return to its natural curves.

THE CHEAT SYSTEM EXERCISE PLAN

There are two major components to the Cheat System Exercise Plan: stretching and exercising. The stretches we showed you earlier in the chapter, but in terms of the "exercising," simply find something that you are excited about doing. Just like most of us view a diet as eating nothing but tasteless lettuce, when a lot of people think of the word *exercise* they think, "Ugh, something boring that I have to do, something hard and difficult and tedious that I just have to get it done somehow."

But, just like a healthy diet doesn't restrict you to eating only tasteless lettuce, the exercises you choose for Cheat System shouldn't be something you hate. Pick something you enjoy, because if you force yourself to do a workout routine that you dislike, it will cause your stress levels to rise, which will defeat the purpose of the exercise you're doing. Find an exercise that you'll look forward to and that you'll actually do, because signing up for a workout you hate is as unsustainable as a restrictive diet—you'll try it for a while and then give up. What you do for exercise doesn't matter nearly as much as actually doing it.

So what should you do? First, appreciate the movement you do all day. I love my bike because riding it doesn't feel like a workout. Hefting a small child all day is a workout. Going to a job in retail, manufacturing, or the service industry where you have to be on your feet all day is a workout. Hauling groceries is a workout. Walking the dog or cleaning the house, both workouts. There are so many ways to work out that don't involve a gym or even sweating.

For instance, I started wearing comfortable shoes or sneakers wherever I could. This is still one of our most popular tips on PEER-trainer. If you don't have to go to work in heels, wear shoes to work that are comfortable to walk in. Your entire day changes depending on whether you can move in what you're wearing.

Another way to work in activity is to pick something active to do with friends and family instead of just making another dinner plan. Shopping is a great one—you don't necessarily have to buy anything, but you'll walk and stand around for a few hours, which is much better for your body than wine and dinner out.

Try to find a sport or activity that you love. Walking, jogging, and running can be great solitary activities or you can find a friend or a group to do it with you. Tennis is great because it stops and starts, which allows you to stay in your baseline; the same applies to skiing, hiking, and most team sports.

If you think of the sports and movement you loved when you were younger those activities are the most often one of the easiest, most sustaining workouts you can do—hiking, walking, baseball, basketball—things where you stop and have breaks or go slow/fast/slow. This kind of exercise is very effective for weight loss.

I DON'T CARE WHAT ACTIVITY YOU DO, SO LONG AS YOU DO IT

IF YOU'RE NOT WORKING OUT NOW . . .

Do alignment exercises every other day.

- **Week One:** exercises 1 through 4
- **Week Two:** exercises 5 through 8
- **Week Three:** exercises 9 through 12

Get twenty minutes of exercise every other day. It's important to exercise twenty minutes total, but it doesn't have to all be at the same time. So, for example you could bike ten minutes in the morning, walk five minutes at lunch, and then play Wii tennis for five minutes in the evening. If every other day is too much for you, exercise at least three times a week.

If you want to, you can do the stretching and the walking more often.

Pick one sport or activity that you love or that you want to try. Use that activity as your workout at least once a week. (Again, if you want to do more, feel free to do more!)

IF YOU'RE ALREADY WORKING OUT . . .

Slow down! You should be able to breathe easily (being able to talk is a good indicator that you're at the right pace), be able to notice your surroundings, and not have to listen to music during your workouts while you're on Cheat System. If you are able to do all of those things—and not feel cravings for sugar and carbs when you're finished—you've done a successful fat-burning workout.

Take one day off your current routine or schedule. If you've been going to spin class four times a week, make it three. If you're running five days a week, make it four. Lengthen your recovery time so your body can make the most of the exercise you've been doing.

Do alignment exercises after your workout to help strengthen your secondary muscle groups. It will help prevent injury.

FOR EVERYONE . . .

Keep in mind that it's okay to huff and puff through 15 percent of your workout. So if you play basketball for thirty minutes, it's okay to be a little winded for a few minutes here and there. When you go for a run, sprinting the last few hundred yards will be great training for races and help you lose weight. (Speeding up or jogging the last few hundred yards of a walk has the same effect.)

Get off the machines at the gym! Though stationery bikes, treadmills, stair climbers, and ellipticals can be great every once in a while, most people zone out because working out on these machines is incredibly boring and repetitive—which puts you in sugar-burning mode more often than not. Try that same workout outside!

Try something different—a new sport, a different class at the gym, or take a walk outside instead of a jog. For example, Zumba is the most incredibly fat-burning workout for someone just starting out.

I know what you're thinking: you've worked out superhard in the past and not lost any weight. And that's superfrustrating. But it is so possible to love exercising. It shouldn't be churn-and-burn. The exercising you do on Cheat System should relax and invigorate you, not stress you out.

ARE YOU EXHAUSTED ALREADY?

If just reading about an exercise plan tires you out, you may have a lot of inflammation in your body. Once you start eating Eats, the inflammation in your body will reduce (see Chapter 2 for more details) and you'll start to have more energy, which will make you feel able to start exercising. You may also be feeling tired and unmotivated because you've been overtraining.

Most of us who love working out (or at least those of us who think it's a necessary thing to do) end up being overtrained at some point. If you're becoming sick frequently, have extra fat around your abdomen (a tummy), or have encountered injuries, big or small, you're probably overtraining.

If you feel tired, unmotivated, sick, or are becoming injured more than normal, scale back your workouts immediately. Recovery is as much a part of working out as exercise is, and you need to build in some recovery time to get back to normal.

Whether you're suffering from inflammation or are just burned out from overtraining, it's best to start small when you do feel up to exercising again. Walk for ten minutes a day instead of fifteen. Start by doing just the stretches, if you have to. I guarantee that if you eat the Cheat System way and get a little more activity in here and there, you'll feel a difference in your energy levels.

PART TWO

3 Weeks, 12 Pounds

CHAPTER 4

The Cheat System Explained

Eats: You Can Never Be Too Rich, Too Thin, or Eat Too Many Eats

Cheats: Keep All the Foods You Love to Eat, Just Limit the Cheats

Finish each day and be done with it. You have done what you could. Some blunders and absurdities no doubt crept in; forget them as soon as you can. Tomorrow is a new day . . .

—RALPH WALDO EMERSON

We've learned from our members' experiences at PEERtrainer that when people start slow, change becomes doable and great things happen. That's why we've created the Cheat System so you can work at your own pace, incorporating the Eats and limiting your Cheats, to get to your goals instead of feeling like you're destined to fail on some regimented, restrictive, all-or-nothing plan.

 "I follow the Cheat System about 80 percent of the time, and keep trying to move closer to the ideal. I feel great when I follow the program closely. I have been doing this for about six months and have lost about fifteen pounds."   —Gail, Plymouth, Michigan

The Cheat Sheet is the key to the Cheat System, and it is very simple. **The Cheat Sheet is a list**—Eats are on the left side and Cheats on the right. (We're going to share the basic list in this chapter, but you also find the Cheat Sheet online at http://www.peertrainer.com/cheat tracker, which we update as we hear from our friends and readers.)

Your number one rule, which you absolutely must follow, is this: You *eat* the Eats. As much as you want. The Eats are the absolute answer, the magic bullet—because when you eat the Eats you gain control over everything else you eat. I really mean that. The Eats keep you full so that when you do eat Cheats—because we all will—you're not going to overdo it or be at the mercy of a ridiculously huge craving.

You've gotta eat the Eats to get rid of those pounds . . . and the more Eats you eat, the more weight you'll lose. So eat, eat, eat, eat, eat, *eat, eat, eat*, **Eat your Eats!**

Now to the part you've all been waiting for: the Cheats. What is a Cheat? A Cheat is food that is listed on the right side of the list, something that isn't going to help you lose weight but that you want, that you really enjoy, or that you crave. On the Cheats System Diet you absolutely are *not* denied. You can eat any food you want, at any time, any place. We've done the work for you so you can eat whatever you want and still lose weight. Eating some Cheat on a regular basis will keep you from developing massive cravings because no foods are off limits. You only count the calories in each Cheat and limit the number of Cheats you have overall throughout the day. Cheating and eating takes nothing off your table. You can still enjoy the foods you love and lose weight.

The Cheat System is simple. It's a list of Eats and Cheats. There's no need to count how much fat, fiber, or sugar is in any food you eat. Eat the Eats and limit your Cheats, plain and simple. Let's begin with the Eats. You get to eat as many Eats as you want at any time. The Eats are unlimited. Don't worry about having a second, third, or fourth serving of any Eats on the list.

You get to eat any food you want in the form of Cheats as well. What exactly is a *Cheat*? A Cheat is the equivalent of 100 calories. It could be 100 calories of cheese, 100 calories of bacon, 100 calories of pizza, a 100-calorie snack pack, 100 calories of whatever. A ½ Cheat (0.5) is equivalent to 50 calories. You don't need to worry about anything other than the number of calories in what you eat of Cheats. We don't measure it any other way. There are no other special exceptions you have to remember. Only that one Cheat = 100 calories. (Well, there is one exception. If it's a zero-calorie filled food or a food that will drive up your cortisol? That's a Cheat, too. There are only a few of these, but I'll explain that later.)

In the beginning, you get 10 Cheats a day. I'm going to outline a full three-week plan for you, and though we'll get into the week-by-week details soon, for now just keep having ten Cheats per day in your mind. Some of you will find it hard to stick to ten Cheats a day, and others will find it easy to eat ten or perhaps even fewer Cheats. I find that when I am "on track" I eat about six Cheats per day. You might be thinking, that's only 600 calories! But keep in mind that I'm eating a significantly higher number than that because I'm eating mostly from the Eats side. I know that no one could be full eating only Cheats; I'm focused on my unlimited Eats. The main focus I want you to have is to maximize your Eats (the left column of the Cheat Sheet) and to keep track of your Cheats (on the right). Eventually, we'll minimize the frequency of Cheats, but you don't have to worry about that right now. Just focus on eating!

"Much easier to follow than other diets/trackers/changes I've tried, especially not having to keep track of every single morsel of food I eat.

"Only keeping track of Cheats is *so* much easier, and I always know I can eat off the free list if I'm hungry without feeling guilty!

"I knew there had to be something more out there than simply counting every single calorie and depriving myself constantly . . . I just couldn't find anything that accomplished that *and* actually fit into my life." —A.J.K., Vallejo, California

It's very simple: Foods are either Eats or Cheats. You can eat as many and as much of the Eats as you want: those foods are unlimited.

You only have to keep track of the Cheats you eat during your day. So you have two columns: foods you can eat unlimited amounts of, and Cheats. When you start the Cheat System in Week One, you get all the Eats you want, but have to stick to ten Cheats each day.

I told you it was simple, right? Well, take a look at the Cheat Sheet chart. Think of this as your menu. You get to eat whatever you want of the Eats, on the left side, in whatever quantities you want. *And* you get to choose ten Cheats of 100 calories each from the right side. (Find the full, continually updated Cheat Sheet at http://www.peertrainer .com/cheattracker.)

THE CHEAT SYSTEM

CHEAT SHEET

THE CHEAT SHEET

Eats on the Left . . .

Vegetables!

An asterisk denotes best bang for your buck: these are full of nutrition and will keep you feeling full, too!

*Artichokes
*Arugula
*Asparagus
 Bamboo Shoots
*Beet greens
 Beets
*Broccoli
*Broccoli rabe
*Brussels sprouts
 Burdock root
*Cabbage, all varieties
 Celeriac
*Cardoon
 Carrots
 Cassava
*Cauliflower
*Celery
*Chayote squash
 Chili peppers
*Collard greens
*Cucumber
 Eggplant
*Endive
*Fiddlehead ferns

 Fennel
*Garlic
*Green beans
*Green onion
*Green peppers
 Jerusalem artichoke
 Jicama
*Kale
 Kohlrabi
*Leeks
*Lettuce
*Mixed greens
*Mushrooms
*Mustard greens
*Okra
 Onions, all kinds,
  including Bermuda,
  red onions, yellow
  onions, white, sweet
 Palm hearts
 Parsnips
*Peas
 Pumpkin
*Purslane

*Radicchio
 Radishes
*Red peppers
 Rhubarb
 Rutabagas
 Salsify
*Scallions
*Seaweed, all varieties
 Shallots
*Snow peas
*Spinach
*Sprouts, all varieties
*Sugar snap peas
*Summer squash
 Sweet peppers
 Sweet potatoes
 Taro
 Tomatoes, all colors
 Turnips
*Watercress
 Winter squash, all
  kinds
 Yams
*Zucchini

Vegetables

White Potatoes

Wheat and Yeast Products

Breads, bagels, etc. (all)
Cakes
Candy
Chips
Chocolate
Cookies
Crackers

Fried foods
Gluten-free products, all kinds
Pasta, all kinds
Pizza
Snacks (including pretzels, low-fat
    bars, granola, and popcorn)

Dairy Products

Butter and all butter substitutes
Buttermilk
Cheese, all kinds
Cream
Crème fraîche
Eggnog

Ice cream
Milk, all cream products
Sour cream
Soymilk
Whipped cream
Yogurt

Eats on the Left . . .

Best Fruits!

Always unlimited and organic is best

Blackberries	Elderberries	Loganberries
Blueberries	Gooseberries	Mulberries
Boysenberries	Grapefruit	Pomegranates
Cranberries	Lemon	Raspberries
Currants	Lime	Strawberries

More Fruit!

Each day your first serving from the list below is an Eat, and after that serving, all fruits become a Cheat.

Apples	Litchis	Plums
Apricots	Longans	Prunes
Bananas	Mangoes	Pummelo
Breadfruit	Mangosteens	Quinces
Cape gooseberries	Melons	Raisins
Cherries	Nectarines	Rambutans
Custard apples	Olives	Sapodilla
Dates	Oranges	Sapote
Figs	Papayas	Soursop
Grapes	Peaches	Starfruit
Guava	Pears	Tamarinds
Jackfruit	Persimmons	Tangerines
Kiwifruit	Pineapple	
Kumquats	Plantains	

Eat Your Beans!

If using canned beans, make sure you rinse the beans, otherwise there is a lot of sodium.

Adzuki beans	Fava beans	Navy beans
Black beans	Great Northern beans	Pigeon peas
Black-eyed peas	Kidney beans	Pinto beans
Cowpeas	Lentils	Red beans
Chickpeas (garbanzos)	Lima beans	Split peas
Cranberry beans	Mung beans	

and Cheats on the Right . . .

Sugars and Sweeteners

Artificial sweeteners, all, including:

Aspartame
  (NutraSweet)
Saccharin
  (Sweet'n Low)

Sucralose (Splenda)
Acesulfame K (Sunett
  or Sweet One)

And natural sweeteners, like:

Brown rice syrup
Honey
Fructose
Corn syrup

Molasses
Beet sugar
Brown sugar
Cane sugar

Coconut sugar
Dextrose
Chocolate, sweets,
  desserts, candy, etc.

An asterisk indicates the best choice for necessary sweeteners.

*Erythritol
*Licorice
*Luo Han Guo

*Sorbitol
*Stevia

*Xylitol
*Yacon syrup

Eats on the Left . . .

Grains and Pseudo-grains

Amaranth	Kañiwa	Teff
Buckwheat	Quinoa	

Good Proteins!

Your first 4-ounce serving at your first meal is an Eat; anything after counts as a Cheat. Try for organic and grass-fed/pastured when you can.

Beef	Pea protein	Sashimi, any kind
Buffalo	Pork (*only* lean cuts of	Shellfish
Chicken	steaks, loins)	Turkey
Egg (two per portion)	Potato protein	Wild game
Fish, wild caught	Rice protein	
Hemp protein	Sacha inchi protein	

Good Fats

Your first serving at your first meal is an Eat; after that it counts as a Cheat.

Almond milk (1 cup)	Coconut milk, canned	Olive oil (1 tablespoon)
Almond butter	(⅙ cup)	Pumpkin seed oil
(1 tablespoon)	Coconut milk, unsweet-	Rice milk
Almonds (6)	ened (1 cup)	Tahini (1½ table-
Almond oil	Coconut oil (1 table-	spoons)
Avocado (⅓ of a large or	spoon)	Walnut oil (1 table-
½ of a small-sized	Flax seed oil	spoon)
avocado)	Goat milk (¼ cup)	High oleic sunflower oil
Buttermilk (¼ cup)	Hemp milk (½ cup)	
Coconut	Macadamia oil	

Nuts and Nut Butters

Still under the category of fats. First serving of 100 calories is an Eat. After that, it counts as a Cheat.

Brazil nuts	Hazelnuts	Pistachios
Cashews	Macadamia	Soy nuts
Filberts	Pecans	Walnuts

Grains

Barley
Bulgur wheat
Cereal
Corn (yes, corn is not a
    vegetable. It's a
    grain)

Millet
Oat bran
Oats
Popcorn
Rice, all kinds
Rye

Sorghum
Spelt
Triticale
Wheat

Proteins

Duck
Liver
Oysters
Veal

Fatty cuts or
    preparation of
    beef and pork
    including:
    Bacon
    Sausage

Soy and
    soy-based
    products,
    all, including:
    Edamame
    Tempeh
    Tofu

Fats

Butter
Canola oil
Corn oil
Cottonseed oil
Ghee

Grapeseed oil
Lard
Margarine
Palm oil
Peanut oil

Safflower oil
Shortening
Soybean oil
Sunflower oil
Vegetable oil

Nuts and Nut Butters

Peanuts

Peanut butter

Eats on the Left . . .

Drinks

Black coffee (after first cup it's a Cheat)
Black tea (after first cup it's a Cheat)
Green tea
Herbal tea
Oolong tea
Water
White tea

Condiments and Spices

These make vegetables taste good!

Allspice
Aniseed
Basil
Bay leaves
Cacao
Capers
Caraway seed
Cardamom
Carob
Cayenne
Celery seed
Chili oil
Cilantro
Cinnamon
Cloves
Coriander seed
Cumin
Curry powder
Dill
Dried chili pepper
Epazote
Fennel seed
Fenugreek
Fish sauce
Garlic
Ginger
Horseradish
Hot sauce
Jalapeño
Juniper berries
Kimchee
Lavender
Lemon
Lemongrass
Licorice
Liquid aminos
Mace
Marjoram
Mint, all kinds
Mustard
Nutmeg
Nutritional yeast
Oregano
Parsley
Peppercorns
Red pepper flakes
Rosemary
Saffron
Sage
Salsa
Sauerkraut
Savory
Salt
Star anise
Thyme
Turmeric
Vanilla
Vinegar, all kinds
Wasabi

The list goes on and on. Take a trip to the spice section for inspiration.

and Cheats on the Right . . .

Drinks

Alcohol
  Beer
  Spirits, all kinds
  Wine
All drinks that have
  added flavors or
  preservatives

Any no-calorie drinks,
  including Crystal
  Light, diet
  sodas. (If you want
  to eat chemicals,
  you'll have to Cheat
  to do it.)

Black coffee and tea
  after your first cup
Gatorade, power
  drinks, mixes
Soft drinks, all

Condiments and Spices

Any kind of spread, dip
Apple sauce
Baba ghanoush
Barbecue sauce
Béarnaise sauce
Chutney
Cocktail sauce
Gravy

Hoisin sauce
Hollandaise sauce
Hummus
Jam
Jelly
Ketchup
Mayonnaise
MSG

Peanut sauce
Plum sauce
Steak sauce
Tartar sauce
Teriyaki sauce
Soy sauce

I want you to think of the Cheat Sheet as a loose framework that teaches you how to eat. I don't want you to get hung up on calories or how you're going to do this every day. You can eat unlimited, unlimited, unlimited amounts of Eats. That's right—you are on a diet, and I am telling you that you can eat as much as you want! You can totally do this, right?

 "I felt that on other diets, I didn't know what I could 'safely' eat, so I restricted myself to a few very low-calorie, low-fat, low-sugar foods to rely completely on. My body was so deprived, I found myself thinking about food constantly. Now I feel that I know what better choices are and I understand that it's okay to eat everything in moderation."
　　　　　　　　　　　　　　　　　—Kendra S., Lawrence, Kansas

Don't Eat the Eats?

A common reaction when some people see the Cheat Sheet for the first time is that they say something like, "But I don't eat any of the Eats!" And that's a really big deal because they'll look at the meals and think, I have to eat salad, I'm screwed. But look further—you don't just eat salad on the Cheat System.

Cheat System Math

Here's what I want you to keep in mind when you prepare a meal:

$$Protein + Fat + Eats = Losing\ Weight$$

What do I mean by that? In every meal, I want you to make sure that you have a traditional protein (chicken, grass-fed beef, fish, two eggs, or lean cuts of beef and pork) or pea/rice protein the size of your palm (usually a scoop or two), roughly a tablespoon of fats, and as many other Eats as you want with Cheats on top. If you focus on the unlimited Eats, I promise you will be full. It can be anything on the Eats list: sautéed kale, artichokes, tomatoes, black beans and salsa or sweet potatoes sprinkled with cinnamon. I don't care what Eats you choose as long as it makes up most of your plate and that you actually eat all of it.

The list is the list—Eats are always free. But you have to limit your Cheats. However, there are always exceptions to the rule!

There are four exceptions to the Cheats. Think of them as "first-serving Eats" more than Cheats. Your first serving of each item listed below is an Eat; then it becomes a Cheat:

1. Your first traditional protein of the day is free (about palm size, 4 ounces of chicken, beef, fish, or 2 eggs or pea/rice or pea/potato protein powder). After the first serving, they are Cheats.
2. Your first fruit of the day (other than the unlimited fruits).
3. Your first healthy fat of the day is free. (1 tablespoon of olive oil, or your first serving of coconut milk as an example).
4. Your first cup of black coffee.

This is what I'd like you to do but I get when you're at a place or an event where you can't—it's okay.

And one other exception? You get to earn Cheats! If you're having a PEERtrainer Cheat System–approved shake, you earn a cheat. You can also earn other Cheats during the three-week plan. More on that later.

VERY IMPORTANT: Yes, beans and the seed grains and sweet potatoes in the Eats list are unlimited. They're unlimited because they're high-nutrient foods and most have fiber. HOWEVER: Have some sense . . . Go with the bang-for-your-buck vegetables as your 80 percent. If you're eating two sweet potatoes every meal (which for me would be virtually impossible because I'd be so full) and you're having trouble losing weight, or you're eating more than half a can of beans at a meal (which again would be really hard with all those greens), you're going to want to limit these.

It's really important to *not portion-control your vegetables*. Eat unlimited quantities! You can't get too much of kale or Swiss chard or broccoli or tomatoes. Forget everything you've ever heard about counting calories and portion control when it comes to vegetables. Eat them, eat them, eat them—as many as you want at every meal. It seems counterintuitive, but it's important. Contrary to what you've probably ever learned about diets before, we've found at PEERtrainer that there is absolutely no reason to portion-control your vegetables, which is why they are unlimited on the Eats list.

A friend recently called me up and said, "Jackie, I love the Cheat System, but I'm hungry on it!" so I asked her what she was eating. She said she was eating chicken breast, and spinach sautéed with olive oil and red pepper flakes (one of my favorites). I asked her the size of the chicken breast, and it was about the size of a deck of cards, so I knew she was eating enough protein for satiation. Then I asked her about how much olive oil she used and she said about a spoonful, so she was getting enough fat. But then I asked about the spinach. She was only eating half a box of frozen spinach—about 5 ounces! No wonder she was hungry! I told her to eat the entire package the next time she made dinner and call me back. She sounded a bit skeptical, but she did what I said. Afterward, when she called me back, she told me she was amazed by how full she felt. *And* as she continues to eat this way, the weight continues to come off!

To be really satisfied, you must eat a traditional or pea/rice protein and a good fat, or you'll end up hungry. And when we are hungry, we tend to make bad choices that makes us feel like we don't have the discipline to follow through on our goal of losing weight. But as I explained earlier, success really isn't about that. It's about making good decisions—which you do when you're not hungry, when you're full and satisfied. That's why the Cheat System Diet works—because it gives your body what it needs to be satiated, and enables you to make the best choices possible.

You need protein and fat to help your body shed weight and to feel full. Remember, if you aren't doing two pounds of vegetables at a meal (and I've only met one person who does this consistently), you'll need the protein and fat. You also need nutrient-rich vegetables to fill you up. And even more important, everything we've been told time and again about portion control and fat and low-fat diets and what have you is rubbish. We have been conditioned to believe that portions of everything matter, when they don't. Only the foods that don't work in our favor, only the Cheats, need to be counted.

I said it once before, but I'll say it again: **Vegetables are the best diet pill because they have tons of nutrients, are low in calories, and** *keep you feeling full.* I have to admit that even I get tripped up sometimes. Sometimes I'm sick of making vegetables or sick of cooking altogether, so I'll just grab whatever's in the refrigerator. I'll eat a piece of chicken and half an avocado, but no veggies because I don't feel like making spinach or a salad. And then I'll be starving one hour later!

"I think the biggest thing [about the Cheat System] is the idea of stuffing myself with vegetables! No portion control on salads or vegetables in general. So I can fill my plate with a colorful and delicious pile of veggies and get completely full, and all that nice fiber keeps me full and satisfied for a long time. Having nutrient-dense food makes *all* the difference."

—Jeanne T., Atlanta, Georgia

I want to give you a real-life example of how the Cheat System math works. Let's say that you decided to make a two-egg omelet for breakfast. The two eggs are your first traditional protein of the day, and the olive oil or butter you cook it in would be the first fat. Remember your exceptions to the rule? So your two-egg omelet is actually Cheat free! But if you only ate two eggs, you'd be hungry. You need to add some Eats to make you full. So you pile on the broccoli, mushrooms, onions, tomatoes, and fresh spinach. Maybe a little basil. And now you're really starting to add in some Eats.

If you decided to have a slice of toast, this is where the Cheats would come in. Each piece of bread is roughly 100 calories, which means you've used just one cheat of the ten you have available in the first week, for breakfast. Now that you've had a filling, healthy meal full of Eats, you will not be hungry until it's time for lunch, and you still have nine Cheats left for the day!

Does that make sense? Ultimately, the ideal Cheat System meal is made up of the same three things: a protein, a fat, and Eats—plus Cheats, if you want.

The only "rules" to cheating properly are:

Eat three meals a day instead of snacking.
Concentrate on what's going to make you full—the Eats.

Even though you are going to be on a diet, while you are doing the Cheat System, you will be fuller than you've ever been in your life—*because* you eat the Eats.

Why Three Meals a Day?

A lot of people freak out when they realize that they will be eating three real meals a day on Cheat System. And I know why: we're addicted to snacking. There are many nutritionists, diet experts, and doctors who recommend frequent, smaller meals. And while that works for some people (athletes especially), it does *not* help you lose weight. The theory goes that if you constantly feed your system, it "burns" calories constantly. But really, what dieticians have found is that eating small, frequent meals actually increases your appetite and the amount of calories you eat, making it harder to lose weight. And though there is some benefit to constantly burning your body's engine, it simply doesn't make up for the extra calories. Three different studies—cited in *The British Journal of Nutrition, Obesity,* and *The American Journal of Nutrition*—have shown that there are no weight-loss benefits to eating small, frequent meals.

Remember how we talked about sugar burning versus fat burning in the chapter on exercise? Eating frequent meals does the exact same thing as the burn-and-churn workout: it keeps you in sugar burning mode. Spacing out your meals encourages the body to enter fat burning mode (even though you're not working out at all!), helping you lose more weight.

What we'd like for you to do is eat three meals a day and entirely avoid snacking if you can. If you have a challenging work and home schedule or have been on a frequent eating schedule (diet or not), you may find that you are starving and have to eat a snack between meals during the first week on Cheat System. I totally get that, and it's okay.

An easy way to "wean" off snacks is to try expanding the time between meals, bit by bit. If you can only last two hours today, aim to space your meals and snacks out by two hours and fifteen minutes. Your body gets used to a routine, just as your brain does, and it needs time to adjust. But, if after a week of trying to space your meals out and you *still* can't go without eating for more than two hours, please see your doctor because you could have a hormonal issue.

Another thing that I want you to try to do is to not eat during the two to three hours before you go to bed. We eat for energy, so eating at that point in the day doesn't really make sense. A lot of us eat before bed as a reaction to our emotions, not because of hunger.

When we are alone with our thoughts, often we turn to food (or to alcohol) to alleviate thinking about deeper issues. That's why most of us drink wine with dinner or eat snacks while watching TV. The slight you feel because your sister chose someone else to talk to instead of you, the kid that's making your son's life hell by teasing him incessantly, your husband's inability to understand your frustrations—for all of these you may turn to cheese and chocolate and cabernet to soothe. If you are one of those people, I have two ways to help you. First, check out the Advanced sections in the next few chapters—each has an emotional component that will help you deal. And second, be sure to eat plenty of Eats during the day—so you're completely full after dinner at night. It will help you say no to the ice cream your partner pulls out of the freezer at 10 P.M.

WINE AFTER WORKING OUT

We all love our wine or alcohol, but a study found that ethanol ingestion after exercise prolonged the increase in cortisol caused by exercise. The cortisol remained elevated by 2 hours. If you work out in the afternoon or evening and then drink wine, that could be the reason you're stressed or feel anxious at night and keeping weight on.

A NOTE ABOUT BREAKFAST

There are many places people make mistakes in terms of diet, but the most common is breakfast. People usually tend to fall in one of two categories:

(1) They skip breakfast hoping to "save" calories for later—which typically results in a binge later on that day;

(2) They have every intention of getting a good start but end up eating dessert for breakfast: you're late to work or dropping off your kids at school, so you grab a whole-grain muffin and a skinny latte. No matter how healthy that sounds—even though it has the words "whole grain" and "skinny" in it, even though you think you're making a little bit better choice—you're still eating dessert for breakfast. And unfortunately, that sets you up for a day of sugar-binge disaster.

Most people are just looking for an easy way to eat something nutritious that tastes good in the five minutes between getting ready for work and heading out the door. It's tough to make a healthy breakfast in the amount of time most of us have, but conventional breakfast food, especially what's commercially available, simply doesn't contain enough Eats. And as you know, the Eats are the diet pill that keeps you full and energized. Since most of us don't have the time to make a full breakfast with tons of Eats, I have a solution.

In Chapter 9, I'm going to teach you how to use quality ingredients to make the best meal replacement shakes. These shakes take less than five minutes to make, use ingredients that are easy to always have on hand, can satisfy your sweet tooth, will wake you up, give you *tons of energy,* and, best of all, fill you up so completely that you won't be hungry until it's time for lunch. You won't be going through sugar withdrawal all morning from that latte and scone, and your tummy won't grumble in your 11 A.M. meeting. *And* you'll lose weight. You won't believe you haven't done this before now. And you'll want to pass it along to everyone because they will be thanking you for months for turning them on to such an easy way to eat a great tasting breakfast and lose weight!

When thinking about how your meals should be eaten throughout the day, I suggest considering switching up the size of your breakfast and dinner, or even switching the actual foods altogether. Dinner can be a small meal like breakfast, and breakfast can be a big meal like dinner. You could have chicken for breakfast and an egg omelet for dinner.

When I suggested to our PEERtrainer community that it was possible to switch up dinner and breakfast, I got a lot of pushback because people just don't have the time. Morning schedules are crazy—you have to get to work, you have to get the kids to school, your husband or partner often needs your help to find his keys or make his breakfast—and I totally get that.

Remember that at every meal, your key is to focus on Eats. Have your "eaties" for breakfast. And lunch and dinner. (And the "cheaties" on the side, as a condiment.)

Do I Have to Be a Gourmet Chef?

Definitely, definitely not! I used to be totally intimidated by cooking. I grew up in a house where people were obsessed with food. During breakfast, we would talk about lunch; at lunch we were talking about dinner. At dinner, we were talking about what we would eat the next day. I felt like I was always talking about food. Dinner was always a big production. Everything revolved around food—if we were going somewhere, we had to figure out where we were going for lunch. By the time I became an adult, I was so completely finished with talking about eating that I completely rejected cooking and food.

I would always think, "Cooking is so much work, why can't I just grab a slice of pizza for a few dollars and move on with my day?" But today I cook. I serve healthy meals to my family that are easy to make. And you can too, even if you are like me and don't particularly love cooking.

However, if you are already a cook, you will enjoy making the recipes on this diet, and experimenting with the recipes you already love. Many of the PEERtrainer members use the Eats list as an ingredient list and shape their recipes around an Eat, later adding in a protein, a fat, and perhaps a Cheat. There's an entire section with recipes called the Cheating Gourmet later in the book (you can find it starting on page 167).

I won't ask you to shop at specialty stores; all the Eats can be found in a normal supermarket. But I am really focused on making healthy food taste good. If you're like me and you don't know the first thing about cooking—even if you don't know how to soak beans or boil an egg—this diet is for you, too.

A lot of diet experts and health gurus tell you that you should prioritize cooking, that you have to learn how to cook in order to eat a healthy diet. And that's simply not true. JJ Virgin, one of our partners, a bestselling diet author and health guru, makes it very well known that she doesn't like to sit in the kitchen cooking. She makes two of her protein and energy shakes to eat as breakfast and lunch, and then makes something really simple like grilled fish and spinach for dinner. No chef skills necessary!

Throughout this chapter, I'm going to give you CheatCuts: little tips and tricks I've discovered on my own or from members at PEERtrainer that make eating healthy super easy. Here's the first one:

I'm going to give you all the things you need to succeed no matter what your abilities or willingness to cook. I've noticed that even the most reluctant cook can make one thing that tastes delicious. And when friends and family fall all over themselves saying how good it is, you think, "Well, that was easy, why don't I try another recipe?" And if the same thing happens, you start thinking "I can do this." And that's how you build

Buy precut and prewashed EVERYTHING. Every grocery has containers of precut produce, prewashed lettuces, mixed greens, even mixes that contain kale, lettuces, arugula, chard, and more. Buy jars of salsa or tomato sauce or premade hummus instead of making your own (just read the label to make sure there aren't any hidden ingredients that you don't want to be eating).

Anything you can get where the prep work has been done for you is well worth buying. Opening packages doesn't require nearly as much effort as becoming your own sous-chef.

your cooking muscles! Some people learn to love cooking, while others (like me) just do it because they have to. Wherever you fall on the spectrum, the Cheat System will work for you.

When I was starting out as a cook and made PEERtrainer Energy Soup (see recipe on page 231), it was easy to lose weight on that soup because it was right there in the fridge. I didn't have to worry about fats or fibers or even Cheats—I could make a meal just by having the soup and adding a protein! It tasted so good and it helped me lose so much weight that people regularly asked me how I did it.

Although I cook lots more now than I did when I started out, I still have limitations. Recently a friend who loves to cook explained to me how she makes her own chicken broth . . . and I have to admit I thought in my head, "That sounds awful." I tried to listen, but I ended up tuning out about halfway through the fifteen complicated steps she was detailing. I thought to myself, "I don't have the time." I felt weighed down just listening to the steps . . . And that's okay! Some people make their own broth and others don't. But both types of people can succeed on Cheat System.

The No-Cook Cheat System Meal

You have to do only three things to have a cooking-free meal with only two Cheats:

1. Go to the grocery store and buy a frozen meal. (Go for organic if you can and make sure the dinner has a traditional protein.) At the same time, buy a pound of frozen spinach, greens, or another Eat you like.

2. When you're ready to eat, remove whatever carbohydrate (rice, pasta) is included in the frozen dinner. (If you want to keep the carbohydrate, that's fine—but count it as Cheats.) Keeping a sauce is okay, or adding your own is fine, too. Then take the frozen Eat and add it on top of the frozen dinner.

3. Heat and serve.

Frequently Asked Questions About Cheating and Eating

Sometimes after people have looked through the list and the Cheat System, they e-mail me to ask questions about why certain foods are Eats while others are Cheats. Here are a few examples of the most commonly asked questions at PEERtrainer:

1. Why are artificial sweeteners Cheats?

Though these products contain very few—or even zero—calories, most are counterproductive to losing weight. Artificial sweeteners like Splenda, Sweet'n Low, and Equal are considered Cheats because of what they do to our bodies and to our behavior.

First, artificial sweeteners are just that: *artificial*. There's not a single natural ingredient in any packet, by any brand. In fact, some ingredients, like aspartame, have been linked in research to the development of cancer. Second, studies have shown that artificial sweeteners actually alter your taste buds, causing you to crave sweeter and sweeter and sweeter foods in order to satisfy the "sweet tooth" you develop by using artificial sweeteners.

And if changing your taste buds isn't scary enough, Dr. Robert Lustig, a pediatric endocrinologist and professor of clinical pediatrics at the University of California San Francisco, explained in his book *Fat Chance* that consuming artificial sweeteners actually causes your body to have the same reaction as it would have if you consumed real sugar—releasing cortisol. But because those artificial sweeteners aren't actually sugar, the cortisol doesn't find any sugar in your blood to process—so it takes sugar from your muscles instead, and most of the time ends up storing that as fat. Even worse, that process inside your body also makes you hungry—which leads to you eating more throughout the day.

That's why I'll never touch a Diet Coke or a packet of Splenda, and why artificial sweeteners are Cheats. Not only are these products full of chemicals, but they'll also cause you to eat more and store more fat!

2. Why is coffee considered a Cheat?

After French fries, coffee is one of our biggest addictions and indulgence. The problem isn't the coffee itself, necessarily: one cup of black coffee in the morning is fine—especially if you choose to work out within forty-five minutes of drinking it. But the problem with coffee is twofold: first, I see people drinking excessive amounts of coffee and not losing weight; and second, most people drink it with tons of cream, milk, and/or sugar—making a low-calorie drink really high in calories and resulting in the same sugar crash as the "dessert for breakfast" example I used earlier.

If you find that you want or need caffeine during the day, drink green tea. It contains powerful antioxidants called catechins that black tea and coffee do not have. These catechins are not only good for your health, but they actually increase fat burning, which is something neither black tea nor coffee can boast!

3. In the exceptions to the rules, why are different Eats that become Cheats (after the first serving) considered equal when many of them have different fat, calorie, and fiber content? For example, 2 eggs are equal to 4 ounces of chicken and those have different nutritional profiles.

Remember, we've done the work for you and we've worked forgiveness into the plan. The focus is on the Eats, not the Cheats. So as long as we've listed something as an Eat (as your first serving) then as a Cheat, it's an Eat, then a Cheat. You can always check at our Cheat Tracker (http://www.peertrainer.com/cheat-tracker) if you're confused and need more information.

4. Do I really earn a Cheat when I have a PEERtrainer Cheat System shake?

Yes, you do! Our shakes do the most important thing: they fill you up and make you feel satisfied with energy. Even if it has a sweetener, if you make our recipe, you earn a full cheat for the day!

5. Can I "bank" my Cheats for a special occasion?

Yes, you can! If you have an event on Saturday, you can have fewer Cheats during the week and save them for the event. You might see the scale go up the next day after the event if you weigh yourself, but it won't be a true number until the following day you've gone right back to your typical Cheat System day.

6. Are there any foods that aren't on the list?

NO. You can eat every food, no matter what. All foods are either a Cheat or an Eat. But it's important to know that all Cheats are not equal. There are some foods we'd prefer that you reduce significantly in your diet or avoid altogether:

+ Smoked foods
+ Processed cold cuts
+ High fructose corn syrup, any sugar substitutes, and other processed chemicals. If you can't pronounce it, you shouldn't eat it. Avoid sugar, processed food, wheat, soy, corn, anything that people have manufactured that hits your satiation point (salt, sugar, and fat), anything that you can't stop eating—basically all junk food, potato chips, candy, etc.—because you will eat and eat and eat those foods. They've spent billions of dollars on marketing, advertising, and chemistry labs to make those foods irresistible—and keep you eating them until the bag is gone.
+ Peanut butter: Whenever you can, swap almonds or walnuts for peanuts.
+ Soy products, including soy milk, soy sauce, and tofu
+ All kinds of wheat
+ Dairy: We know many of you will ask about calcium. But you will diversify your sources of calcium by eating green vegetables. These foods are packed with calcium, and other nutrients your body needs to absorb it.
+ An overwhelming amount of fruit (though your first fruit of the day is free)

The reason I ask you to reduce your intake of these Cheats in particular is because I want you to get results. After years of studying our members at PEERtrainer, I created this list very carefully and strategically. If you increase the amount of vegetables and decrease processed foods and chemicals you eat, your body simply runs better.

I can't say it enough: eat your Eats, especially vegetables, vegetables, vegetables. One thing we've learned at PEERtrainer is that there is a strong correlation between health and weight loss. Here's the secret: it takes time to get your health back in order. People abuse their bodies for twenty-five years and think they can go on a six-week natural health cleanse and all will be well. This is not the case. You will definitely lose your ten pounds in three weeks, but your health goals should be something you stick to, not something you fail at and then feel bad about yourself. Being on the Cheat System will get you results both in the short term for your weight and in the long term for your overall health.

As part of that, I want you to think differently about every meal. Instead of thinking, "We're having roast beef tonight; what vegetable should we have on the side?", we want you to think, "What vegetables are we having for dinner, with roast beef (Cheats!) on the side?" Change how you think about sandwiches. Bread isn't necessary most of the time; you can eat chicken salad as part of a bigger greens salad instead of automatically putting it between slices of bread. Think of the Cheats as your "side" dish and the Eats as your "main" dish or as the entrée.

As you start to increase your vegetable consumption you'll probably start to find that you actually eat fewer than ten Cheats a day. Why? Because you'll be so satisfied from the high-nutrient foods you're eating from the left side of the menu that you simply won't need to eat as much from the Eats.

The more you increase your Eats and decrease Cheats, the quicker you'll see the numbers on your scale go down. In other words, focusing on the fact that you can eat unlimited Eats won't make you feel limited by your weekly number of Cheats.

WILL THIS WORK FOR GUYS?

Yes. If you're a big guy and are very active you may find yourself adding a few Cheats if you're still hungry eating only ten per day. With extra Cheats, your weight may drop a bit slower, but you'll have to figure out what works best for your body and energy level. Some men find that when they are in the groove, they eat fewer than ten Cheats on most days because their staples are Eats: sweet potatoes, beans, vegetables, seeds, nuts, and various soups. This is what gives great energy all day, and keeps even "insane man hunger" satisfied. If you're an athlete, please go to page 329 in the appendix for more information about the Cheat System for athletes.

Cheating and Eating Out

Here's the truth about Cheat System, from someone who's actually been on it and been successful: I don't say no to anything, and you shouldn't either. **You should feel free to use Cheats as you want to.** You can save up Cheats over the course of a day or even the course of a week and splurge on a particular meal, or you can use a Cheat or two at every meal. Personally, I find it easier to use Cheats in bunches because it's easier to keep track of that way—but you should do what works for you.

For example, you can save your Cheats up for a special occasion or happy hour. If you're eating the Eats most of the time, your body or weight won't be all that affected by one happy hour or meal out. I go many days using only six Cheats per day because I'm eating the Eats and feel full. I save up Cheats so that I *can* go crazy when I am eating out every once in a while. On those occasions, I enjoy anything I want and I don't gain weight.

 "I really enjoy that on the Cheat System there is nothing that you can't eat. You can eat any 'bad' or 'unhealthy' food as long as it's in moderation. Somehow, knowing that helps me have more motivation to eat good foods."
—Sara, Texas

Eating out is actually *why* I developed the Cheat System the way I did. You don't have to stress out at a restaurant and worry about preparation, fat, fiber, or calories. You just have to know what is a Cheat and how many of them you have. You don't have to stop going out to eat with your friends; you don't have to mentally prepare for dinner with your spouse or try to be psychologically strong around your coworkers when they invite you out to celebrate someone's promotion.

GUARD YOUR MIND

As you begin to progress and lose weight, people will say things to you. Often these are negative, counterproductive statements; sometimes people can be downright hurtful. These are times when you should guard your mind. I like to picture the big steel gates of a fortress. When someone begins to criticize me for how I'm eating, or questions why I'm doing something I'm doing, I close my gates. I put mental space between myself and their negativity so it won't affect me (or at least not as much). This is a great tactic to use when you find that other tactics you've learned aren't enough.

Losing weight is not whether we're capable of being psychologically strong; we are. But we all need flexibility in our lives. People are complicated and contradictory—it's just part of human nature. On the Cheat System, we accept that. We stop beating ourselves up on the Cheat System for eating chocolate or French fries. The fact is, you're going to eat cheese and crackers once in a while, but it's not the end of the world and you can still lose weight!

When I accepted that life happens, I knew that the Cheat Sheet and the Cheat System are designed to work in real life by teaching you to accept the fact that you're going to make mistakes, but that it's okay—and that even if you cheat on your diet, you will still lose weight.

It's very easy to eat out and be social on Cheat System: wherever you go, you just need to estimate what the Cheats are. Look at your plate: other than a palm-sized portion of protein, a cherry tomato of fat, and all of your Eats, everything else is a Cheat. As you get more familiar with counting your Cheats, you'll have a rough notion of how many Cheats something is. For example, a slice of bread is usually around one Cheat. A restaurant serving of pasta, especially with the sauce, is usually five or six Cheats.

A Sushi Substitute

Try an interesting experiment. If you're the type of person who gains weight when you eat Japanese, Chinese, or Thai food, the reason might be because of the soy sauce.

Instead of soy sauce, lemon is a great substitute. At sushi restaurants, squeeze a quartered lemon in the small soy sauce dish and mix it with a bit of wasabi. And don't worry about asking for it: most restaurants keep slices of lemon on hand for people who like it in green tea.

When you're eating out, it's almost always safe to order a salad or an appetizer with a side portion of vegetables as your side. Restaurants typically do a terrific job of preparing vegetables, and ordering these sides is the best way to get nutrients in without having to cook. Whether it's broccoli rabe at an Italian restaurant (a great substitute for pasta), baby green spinach at an American restaurant, or sautéed vegetables at a Thai restaurant, professional chefs create inventive flavor combinations and preparations for Eats out. In fact, you may even be able to learn a thing or two by ordering vegetable sides from restaurants. However, be sure to ask for light on the oil and salt and heavy on the spices!

Ordering a traditional dinner entrée is dangerous because the portion sizes tend to be huge! Even if you ordered a salad—especially something that depends on the dressing or cheese to make it tasty, like a Caesar salad—the amount of Cheats in a restaurant portion is usually double if not triple the number of Cheats if you were to make that same salad at home.

And don't tell me that you're going to order the entrée and only eat half of it, because more often than not, you don't. Be honest with yourself—you'll probably eat the entire thing. Don't do it. Instead, go for a side of vegetables and your favorite appetizer. You'll leave just as full, but with more Cheats to use another day.

A very easy way to limit your Cheats while dining out is to treat everything that's not an Eat like a condiment. Treat Cheats like you would treat ketchup or mustard or mayo in any other situation. You wouldn't eat an entire plate of ketchup, right? Whether it's a slice of bread or a pat of butter, treat it like a condiment and usually you'll only use a single Cheat.

If you're out and don't want to order a salad, feel free to follow the appetizer-and-side rule. But if you do, that can be a great way to experience a new way of preparing Eats. Personally, I love that someone else is making that salad for me! It's like a dream that someone else is going to fix my yummy salad. A while back, I had the best salad made for me at a restaurant. It had pine nuts, red onions, mixed greens, chicken, and this delicious lime vinaigrette. (And that recipe, from the Mediterranean Restaurant in Boulder, Colorado, is in the recipe section on page 203! You must try it if you love to cook.)

PICK YOUR PLEASURE: WINE, BREAD, OR DESSERT

When you go out to eat, you're not going to have just a little bit of bread or a little bit of wine or a little bit of dessert. If you go crazy once in a while, that's okay, but if you're anything like me and you end up eating out more than you'd like—I have to eat out for a lot of business lunches, and my husband likes going out to dinner together—you need to know how to handle it.

Sometimes I look at what other people order and it's mouthwatering. My husband recently ordered steak frites—it was a beautiful steak, topped with gorgonzola, with French fries on the side. I end up being at the same table as food like that pretty frequently—and so I decided I had to *pick my pleasure.*

Your pleasure, whether it's wine, bread, or dessert, will still be a Cheat. But going a little overboard on one is certainly better than going overboard on all three. Personally, I tend to pick wine or the dessert because bread just isn't worth it for me. But what you pick is up to you.

I decided on the "pick your pleasure" idea because I used to have a three-bite rule at dessert (you could order any dessert you want but you could have only three bites), and then I realized that when you order and taste dessert, you're going to eat the whole thing, period. This way, you go overboard on only one thing—not everything.

Habit-Forming Habits

It's important to remember, now that you're about to try the Cheat System and change the way you eat, that you'll also be changing your habits. And typically, habits are paired: for instance, your morning coffee might be paired with a piece of toast.

If coffee and a cinnamon roll is a habit you have—especially if you've had it for years—you will find that trying to have a cup of coffee without that cinnamon roll will be really hard. When you start the Cheat System, it will be easy to examine what hook-on habits you have by figuring out what foods you really crave on the Cheat list. There can good hook-on habits (I put my gym clothes in my car, so I have them when I go to work out). But there are a ton of food-related ones, most of which are really bad. For example, even years after I stopped eating this way, it's still really hard for me to have a bacon, egg, and cheese sandwich without a huge cup of coffee with lots of sugar and cream. It's an old habit, and an outdated habit for me, but still, it exists. Most of us have these habits that we don't even realize, because they are so ingrained. And they multiply: a hook-on habit can have two elements like the ones I mentioned above, or three elements or even four. Let's say you go to your favorite Italian restaurant, where you used to always eat the bread, the pasta, and the tiramisu. The moment your brain tastes a bite of that bread, you're likely to order the pasta and you're definitely going to have the tiramisu for dessert.

Now that I'm aware of my own hook-on habits, I try to avoid anything that's part of a hook-on habit for me unless it's a good habit. For example, I live for my Tex-Mex Salad (recipe on page 208) because it has potato chips and it's crunchy and delicious. But for whatever reason, I drank green tea with that salad the first few times I made it. So now every single time I set out to make that salad, I have to make green tea. I can't have that salad without that green tea—which is not a bad habit in the least!

One of our members recently wrote in about her favorite hook-on habit:

"Every morning when I get up, I make a cup of black coffee. I get ready while I'm drinking it, so that the minute the empty cup is in the dishwasher, I'm out the door—to walk my dog, to go for a run, or to go work out at the gym. It's become such an ingrained habit that I even do it on vacation!"   —Meghan S., New York City

This Is Not "Diet" Food

I want you to stop eating "substitution foods." What I mean by that is eating a turkey burger and sweet potato fries when you really want a burger and fries, or substituting some kind of weird health-food pizza with brown-rice crust or whole wheat crust for a normal pie. All of those concoctions—and they are concoctions—don't replace the emotional yummy taste you're going for. Often once you're done with its substitution, you're going to still want the pizza or the burger—and then you've doubled the calories of that craving! Save your Cheats for things you really want, not for substitute concoctions. The trend of "let's have quinoa pizza" rarely works because it tastes like cardboard and you still want real pizza after anyway.

"Other diets kept me eating the same fat-free sugar-free 'fake' foods every day because I was too afraid to venture. Not so much anymore. Now I can freely experiment with the flavors of real food. Food tastes better now that I don't eat sugar or sugar substitutes (post-cleanse). I was missing a lot." —Heather, New York City

Change the focus to the Eats. Substituting "healthy" concoctions for what you really want isn't satisfying. Figuring out which artificial sweetener might be better for you is a waste of time. Sure, some sweeteners are better than others, but at the end of the day, it doesn't matter whether agave is better than Splenda because it's all sugar, it all lacks micronutrients, and it's all Cheats.

 "Honestly, the Cheat System is the best thing you have given me so far. I followed it very extensively for a month and now it has become a template for how I eat. It helped me plan for when I wanted something sweet. It was really easy to determine how many calories I was really consuming and where to make allowances for treats. It made it so easy and now no food has to be off limits. It gave me choices but still keeps me in control of where I like to be." —Kimberly, San Antonio, Texas

The Cheat System combines the greatest diet tools out there: it's a high-nutrient lifestyle that also allows for cookies and desserts (the real, whole-fat ones). A nutrient-rich lifestyle is the only path toward health, but we need that path to have forgiveness, which is what the Cheat System is. If you eat your Eats you won't have to worry about eating quinoa pizza or arguing about honey and agave because those will be Cheats and you'll be okay eating those foods occasionally—nutritionally and in terms of your weight.

Once I created the Cheat System and introduced it to our PEERtrainer community, people loved it. As I mentioned in the introduction, more than 100,000 people downloaded and/or shared our original guide to the Cheat System. In an ongoing survey, our members lost an average of 14.2 pounds over three months. But many asked for a more detailed plan—specifically a week-by-week plan that gave them ideas for meals, more structure, and helpful information.

So we created the three-week Cheat System diet plan that's in this book. I created meal plans with easy recipes to go along with the list. Each of the next three chapters covers one week of the twenty-one days that are going to change the way you eat, how you feel, and what size you wear. What you'll learn in those chapters will help you lose up to twelve pounds in just three weeks!

Are you ready to start cheating and eating?

CHAPTER 5

Cheat System Plan Week One

Eat the Eats, and You Have 10 Cheats

This week, I want you to **focus on the Eats.** Try to incorporate as many as you can. Eat as many Eats as you want; **Eats are unlimited, so eat as much as you want! If you're still hungry when you finish your first plate of Eats, go for a second!**

Calories are not created equal. The nutrients in the Eats from the Cheat Sheet will give you the nutrients you need to stay satiated and full until your next meal. That's the reason those Eats are completely unlimited. The portions for the traditional protein (about the size of a deck of cards or of your palm) and the fat (a tablespoon or a cherry-tomato-sized dollop) are somewhat set because those aren't strictly nutrient based.

Your body will use the high micronutrients in the food you eat—it's what we at PEERtrainer call "eating for energy." If you eat the Cheat System way, you'll still be full and have energy for hours afterward, because your body's levels of cortisol and blood sugar are completely stable. You won't be hungry for hours because you'll have eaten the micronutrients and vitamins your body craves. Simply put, you'll be amazed at how you feel. I did not really understand myself how eating for energy and for my body worked until I began having a high-nutrient lifestyle and started being conscious of Cheats. I avoided being tired at

11 A.M. and 2 P.M.—I had energy all day to do the things I needed to do. The change in what I was eating made all the difference.

Don't know if something is an Eat or a Cheat? Check out the always updated list at http://www.peertrainer.com/cheattracker and if you *still* don't find it, e-mail us!

But remember, the **10 Cheats** you can eat every day this week are there for a reason. First, you're going to need to cheat because your body and your mind will want the Cheats. *And* you'll lose weight even while eating that many Cheats each day this week.

However, if you eat more than the Cheats allotted for each day or the week, you won't be following the Cheat System—you can't cheat all the time and lose weight, period.

Before you check out our sample meal plans, I want you to keep these five things in mind:

1. Get rid of your junk.

Take the issue of discipline or of willpower out of the picture. You can't eat what you don't have in your home.

2. When in doubt, Vegetables + Protein + Fat = Lose Weight

When you're thinking about what to eat at any time of the day, this should be your guide. Remember what a Cheat System meal looks like: a palm-sized or deck-of-cards-sized portion of traditional protein, a tablespoon or cherry-tomato-sized portion of fat, and at least a grapefruit-sized portion of vegetables—and as many additional vegetables as you want (and Cheats on top!).

3. You don't have to *make* anything!

Don't feel like cooking? Not up for washing lettuce? Grab a cucumber and sprinkle some salt. Tomatoes are great for that as well. Don't worry about recipes if cooking isn't your thing. Many times I put together the strangest combinations because it's easy and it's what appealed to me at the moment.

4. But if you do cook, rotating through meals you love is fine!

Eating the Cheat System way should not feel like prison. Find three or four meals that you love, savor, and look forward to and are psyched about. This week, I want you to focus on finding these three or four meals that taste good and give you energy. Put them into standard rotation and make them meals you can rely on to satisfy you in a healthy way. When you feel like experimenting you can—but these will be your standbys.

5. Buy high-quality fish oil capsules.

It's like a booster. Good fat helps your body burn fat—and it detoxifies. Fish oil capsules contain "good" omega-3 fats, which help your body reduce belly fat. That's why we include taking them on a daily basis on the Cheat System. Fish oil is like a diet booster because the "good" omega-3 fat it contains helps your body burn more fat and detoxifies your body.

Look for a high-quality brand that offers 500 to 1,000 milligrams combined EPA and DHA per capsule, and try to get a total of 2 to 4 grams EPA/DHA every day. If you are currently taking blood-thinning medication, make sure to see a doctor first!

FOCUS ON THE EATS, BUT . . .

Remember that diet is only 75 percent of what goes into the losing weight—and the other 25 percent comes from getting your body moving. So remember what we discussed in Chapter 3: that ideally I'd like for you to walk for twenty minutes every other day. But it doesn't have to be all at once; you can take a five-minute walk in the morning, a ten-minute walk after or before lunch, and a five-minute walk after work. I don't care how the twenty minutes happens, just that it does.

On the days you're not walking, you should do the Egoscue alignment stretches in Chapter 3. The combination will help keep your body in balance.

And if you're freaking out about doing a shorter workout, it's okay to do what you've been doing—just be sure to *slow it down.* It will help you get off the sugar-burning treadmill you've been on, reduce the cortisol in your body, and help you get in fat-burning mode.

You will see results if you combine the Cheat System way of eating with the Cheat System way of exercising. The combination is key; the only thing I dislike hearing more than "I'm just going to diet, I don't need to work out" is "I'm going to lose weight by hitting the gym and not by changing my eating!" You need to do *both*—that's why both exercise and high-nutrient eating are mandatory parts of our plan.

I don't ask that you work out for hours at a time or that you work out every day—but that just that you do *something.* If you don't move your body, regardless of how well you're eating, you simply won't see the same results.

CHEAT WEEK ONE MEAL PLAN

This is going to be easy. **I don't want you to get hung up on what the meal plans here look like.** What I do want you get hung up on is that unless you eat from the Eats category, you're limited to 1,000 calories of Cheats per day and no one can survive on that. *You must eat your Eats.*

Treat the meal plans as guidance and inspiration, not as rules to follow. Feel free to mix and match. These are simply meant to show you how Cheating and Eating works—and how delicious it can be.

You can find all of our recipes in Chapter 9, starting on page 167—and there are thousands more on http://www.peertrainer.com /cheattracker, being updated all the time!

Week One Meal Plan

Day 1

> Breakfast: 2 eggs scrambled with 1 slice bacon, mushroom, and spinach; half grapefruit; piping hot cup of raspberry or green tea, or one cup of black coffee
>
> Total Cheats: 1—from the bacon. Remember, your first serving of protein here is free (as is the olive oil you used to prepare the omelet with; it's your healthy fat!).

LUNCH: Weight-Loss Shortcut Soup (2 servings) with Easy Foil Rosemary Chicken (4 ounces); bring a thermos!

Total Cheats: 3—from coconut milk in soup (2) and chicken (1)

EATING OUT: Chipotle Bowl with palm-sized chicken, pico de gallo and salsa, palm-sized beans, golf-sized portion of guacamole

Total Cheats: 3—from the chicken (2) and guacamole (1)

DINNER: Hot Italian Salmon Garlic Scampi with a large bed of chopped romaine and Creamy Caesar Salad Dressing; one 5-ounce glass of cabernet or chardonnay

Total Cheats: 4.5—2 tablespoons of the salad dressing (1), salmon (2), and wine (1.5)

Cheats: You've used 8.5 Cheats. You have 1.5 remaining.

Day 2

BREAKFAST: Chocolate Almond Sea Salt Shake. You may also add 8 ounces of black coffee to this shake if you're having trouble giving up the sugar or cream in the coffee.

Total Cheats: 0 (Free! Because of the exceptions to the Cheat rule.)

LUNCH: Di's Hot Sausage Spice Soup (1 portion, 1 Cheat) and Savory Rosemary Chicken Salad

Total Cheats: 3—from the sausage, chicken, avocado, and oil

DINNER: Shrimp Taco Wraps with Black Beans and salsa (2 servings)

Total Cheats: 3—from shrimp and avocado

Cheats: You've used 6 Cheats. You have 4 remaining.

Day 3

BREAKFAST: Scott's Summer Breakfast Salad with 2 hard-boiled eggs; 1 cup of hot tea or 1 cup of coffee

Total Cheats: 0—your first protein, piece of fruit, healthy fat, and cup of coffee is free!

Lunch: Avocado and Bacon Chicken Salad on a large bed of mixed greens
Total Cheats: 3—from the chicken and the bacon
OR
Di's Hot Sausage Spice Soup and Savory Rosemary Chicken Salad (leftovers)!

Eating out: Subway Grilled Chicken Salad with 1 slice of bacon—load up on the greens! Balsamic vinaigrette (1 tablespoon)
Total Cheats: 3—from the chicken and dressing

Snack: Apple with ½ tablespoon almond butter; 1 cup of green tea
Total Cheats: 2—from the apple and almond butter

Dinner: Spring Fresh Cherry-Tomato Appetizer; Insane Man Hunger Chili (2 servings)
Total Cheats: 3—from the oil and beef

Cheats : You've used 8.5 Cheats. You have 1.5 remaining.

Day 4

Breakfast: Brian's Mint Chocolate Chip Cookie Smoothie
Total Cheats: 0—This is a PEERtrainer-approved shake and your first serving!

Lunch: Asian Chicken Salad
Total Cheats: 2

Eating out: Large bed of mixed greens; 1 tablespoon of olive oil and freshly squeezed lemon; 4 ounces of whatever grilled protein is available at the restaurant
Total Cheats: 2 from the protein and dressing

Dinner: Brian's Sweet Potato and Coconut Meatballs with tomato sauce (2 Cheats) (1 serving); Garlicky Mashed "Pota-

toes" (1); Roasted Broccoli with Cheat Confetti Parmesan Crisps (1.5); PEERtrainer Pumpkin Pie (1)
Total Cheats: 5.5

Cheats: You've used 7.5 Cheats. You have 2.5 remaining.

Day 5

BREAKFAST: Triple Berry Smoothie (or a shake from the breakfast recipe section)
Total Cheats: 0—This is a PEERtrainer-approved shake and your first serving!

LUNCH: Slow-Cooker Chicken and Spinach Soup; Perfect Sweet Potato Fries
Total Cheats: 3—for the bacon, coconut milk, and chicken

DINNER: Spicy Thai Curry (2 servings with a cup of rice) (3 Cheats); one 5-ounce glass of cabernet or 1.5 Cheats worth of dark chocolate
Total Cheats: 4.5

Cheats: You've used 7.5 Cheats. You have 2.5 remaining.

Day 6

BREAKFAST: Chocolate Raspberry Torte Shake
Total Cheats: 0!

LUNCH: Tex-Mex Salad with Potato Chips
Total Cheats: 2.5—from the avocado and potato chips

DINNER: Warm Cream of Tomato Soup and Classic Italian Grilled Cheese (5 Cheats); Simple Sautéed Spinach; Garlicky Mashed "Potatoes" (1)
Total Cheats: 6 —from the coconut milk, bread, butter, cheese, and avocado

Cheats: You've used 8.5 Cheats. You have 1.5 remaining.

Day 7

BREAKFAST: Meg's Mexican Breakfast Skillet (2 Cheats)
Total Cheats: 0 (first protein and fat are free!)

LUNCH: Italian Herb Goddess Chicken OR 4 ounces of tilapia
OR a lean cut of chicken or grass-fed beef (1.5 Cheats); The Fa-
mous Puréed PEERtrainer Energy Soup (1 serving) (1 Cheat)
Total Cheats: 2.5

DINNER: Chicken, Artichoke, Mushroom, with Parmesan Casserole (2 Cheats); Brussels Sprouts with Bacon (1 Cheat)
Total Cheats: 3—from the chicken, parmesan, oil, and bacon

Cheats: You've used 5.5 Cheats. You have 4.5 remaining.

Remember, you don't have to "cook" and make all of these recipes—
you can put a few recipes into rotation instead. I cook only a couple of
days a week, but I know my plate. Your plate should look like this:

+ One 4-ounce serving of traditional protein or pea/rice protein
+ 1 tablespoon of a healthy fat
+ Tons of Eats! Fill your plate! Fill it again!

And the rest are Cheats.

THE CHEAT INCENTIVES

Each week, I'll challenge you to do a mental and a physical activity. These aren't
hard, but what I'm asking you to do might be out of your comfort zone. I urge
you to try each and every one—not just because you earn free Cheats, but
because these are proven to help you lose more weight.

The Week One Cheat Incentives are:

• You can earn **one extra Cheat this week** if you follow the Cheat System
Exercise Plan (below) for Week One, try a new sport, or participate in an
activity you loved as a child.

- You can earn **two extra Cheats this week** by taking care of actions you have been putting off. These could be little things, like fixing something broken in your home, or big things like telling a friend that she hurt your feelings. Write each action down on a list, and when you're done, cross it off. The list can be handwritten, on your computer, or in the notes section on your phone (which is what I do). It just has to be somewhere outside your own thoughts. When you're done with each action—and not before—you earn one Cheat for the week. (If you complete both actions, you earn two.)

Week One to Do

+ Weigh yourself and record your weight. I'd like you to weigh yourself every day or at least once a week. You can't finish the marathon if you don't know where your start line is. We have a home for you to do this at http://www.peertrainer.com/cheattracker.

+ Include your goal. It doesn't matter what your goal is, but I want you to have one and write it down.

Week One Exercise Plan

+ Do the Egoscue Exercises 1 to 4 every other day (it takes only 10 minutes!).

+ Be active for 20 minutes total every other day. The time can be broken up however you want; you can spend 20 minutes walking, or just 5 minutes walking and 15 minutes playing Wii Tennis, or 10 minutes walking the dog twice a day. Just get in your 20 minutes.

CHAPTER 6

Cheat System Plan Week Two

Eat the Eats and Earn More Cheats

By now, you should be getting used to how cheating and eating works. This week I'm going to ask you to keep eating your Eats but limit your Cheats to eight instead of ten. So each day this week, you will be able to eat **eight Cheats**—*but* you have an opportunity to earn **two more** each day this week through both the mental and physical Cheat incentives (at the end of this chapter), but also through eating seeds and greens.

So what do you have to eat to get those extra Cheats?

1. Get an extra half Cheat each day by eating 1 tablespoon of flax or chia seeds.

Though chia and flax seeds come from different plants, both have huge health benefits. Full of protein, fiber, and omega-3 "good" fat, these small seeds are nutritional powerhouses, keeping you full and fighting inflammation.

Both chia and flax seeds are great in shakes, but make sure to add these seeds last to a shake, so the mixture doesn't get thick. You can also sprinkle them over salads and soups or include them in your green tapenade.

2. Get one full extra Cheat each day by eating an extra ½ pound of greens after 5 P.M.

A quick reminder of what "greens" means: kale, spinach, collard greens, mustard greens, romaine lettuce, mixed greens, Swiss chard, arugula. Check the Cheat Sheet for more.

Remember **you can earn only 1.5 Cheats total each day.** So you can't eat chia and flax seed for every meal in order to get six extra Cheats; that's not how it works (though if you want to eat that much chia and flax, good for you). It simply means that if you do either of those two things—or eat extra greens in the evening—you'll get one Cheat, and if you have the chia, you will earn an extra half Cheat each day.

I recently saw a message on our Facebook wall that said, "How could a half a pound of vegetables negate the chocolate I wanted?"

I asked our Facebook friend what she meant, and whether she ate the half pound of vegetables. She had—she ate a half a pound of spinach, some broccoli, a serving of cod, and a glass of wine. But by eating the extra greens she earned an extra Cheat—she *could* have a one-Cheat-sized portion of chocolate if she had wanted. But she didn't—because she was full!

And that's the reason it's the incentive for the week. Greens are the best diet pill available, and will have more impact on your weight than any Cheat you "earn" by eating it. Remember the three stomachs from Dr. Joel Fuhrman in Chapter 2? The experience this member had is the perfect example of this concept—she ate so many greens she was completely satiated, full, and couldn't even eat her Cheat if she wanted to. Of course she can eat her Cheat another time, and that's fine, too!

In this week's meal plan, you'll notice recipes for our PEERtrainer soups and shakes. All are easy to make, and I want you to make one of each this week.

Week Two CheatCut

Use a food processor to chop greens up into a "green tapenade." It almost seems like you've chopped tons of herbs in your salad. It's a great way to add the extra half pound of greens to earn the extra Cheat each day! You can put it on top of salads or in soups, or warm it up and put it on top of your traditional protein.

"The *most* helpful aspect was the recipes, since I simply didn't know how to cook differently. It is easier to cook this way. I just made up a recipe box with only your recipes. I will use this all summer!"

—Scott, New York City

The shakes are a meal on their own, but if you choose to make a soup, pair it with a traditional protein for a full meal. If a soup seems intimidating to you, try making a shake—it takes only a few minutes.

CHEAT WEEK TWO MEAL PLAN

+ Eat your Eats. You have 8 Cheats per day.
+ Keep taking your 2 to 4 milligrams EPA/DHA from fish oil capsules every day!
+ You can earn an extra half Cheat for eating 1 tablespoon of chia or flax seeds.
+ You can earn one extra Cheat for eating ½ pound of greens after 5 P.M.
+ Try a shake or a soup this week.

Remember, following the meal plans are optional. Feel free to mix and match recipes from this meal plan with what's in Chapter 9. If all you want to do one night is add some greens to a frozen dinner, that can be a great Cheat-free meal!

This might seem weird, but Swiss chard and spinach are the perfect ingredients to add to our shakes! Neither changes the taste of a recipe *at all* and both provide nutrients you need to feel full. And remember, you earn an extra Cheat.

Week Two Meal Plan

Day 1

BREAKFAST: Chocolate Decadence Shake
    with a cup of black coffee
Total Cheats: 0 cheats!

LUNCH: Creamy Chicken Salad with ⅓ of

an avocado; 1 tablespoon chia seeds (the seeds are optional, but you'll earn an extra ½ Cheat if you do!); 5 handfuls of chopped mixed greens; sliced tomato sprinkled with sea salt

Total Cheats: 2.5 (only 2 if you used chia seeds)

DINNER: Tangy Tenderloin (3 cheats); sweet potato sprinkled with cinnamon; 1 pound of Simply Sautéed Spinach (extra Cheat for the extra half pound!)

Total Cheats: Only 2 if you actually make the pound of spinach; 3 if not

DESSERT: PEERtrainer Pumpkin Pie

Total Cheats: 1—from the sugar and coconut oil

Cheats: You've used 5 Cheats. You have 3 remaining if you followed the incentives. If not, you've used 6 to 6.5 Cheats and you have 1 to 1.5 remaining.

Day 2

BREAKFAST: Mango Lassi Shake

Total Cheats: 0! (Remember, PEERtrainer-approved shakes are free)

LUNCH: Tequila-Pineapple Dressing on mixed greens (0.5 Cheats); Mexican City Chicken Salad with ½ cup of black beans (1.5 Cheats)

Total Cheats: 2—from the pineapple, avocado, and chicken

DINNER: Mint and Shallot Halibut with Kale and Oven-Roasted Tomatoes (or large salad with extra kale on the side)

Total Cheats: 1.5—from the halibut and oil

COCKTAIL: Muscle Recovery Margaritas (or Virgin!)

Total Cheats: 2—from the tequila

Cheats: If you had the margarita, you've used 5.5 Cheats and have 2.5 remaining. If you have a Virgin margarita, you only used 3.5 Cheats and have 4.5 remaining.

Day 3

BREAKFAST: Leftover halibut with the Power Workout Breakfast for a powerful day! OR simple 2-egg omelet with your favorite vegetables
Total Cheats: 0!

LUNCH: Chicken with Peruvian Green Sauce (2 Cheats); large mixed greens with Green-Tea Poppy Seed Mint Vinaigrette (1 Cheat)
Total Cheats: 3—from the chicken, oil, and orange juice

DINNER: Easy Italian Herb Baked Turkey (1 Cheats); The Famous Puréed PEERtrainer Energy Soup (1 Cheat); 1 pound of sautéed swiss chard
Total Cheats: 2—from the meat and coconut milk

DESSERT: Easiest Apple Cinnamon Dessert OR apple cored with honey, ½ teaspoon of butter, a dash of cinnamon, microwaved for 60 seconds
Total Cheats: 1 (your first fruit is free!)

Cheats: You've used 6 Cheats for the day. You have 2 remaining (3 if you had the full pound of sautéed swiss chard).

Day 4

BREAKFAST: Two hard-boiled eggs; ½ sliced tomato and cucumber or fresh berries; ½ grapefruit; 1 cup of coffee (black)
Total Cheats: 0!

LUNCH: Spinach salad with Watermelon-Mint-Caper Dressing (0 Cheats) and 1 tablespoon of chia seeds; Orr's Island Vegetable Soup (0 Cheat); 4 ounces of chicken breast (1.5 Cheats)
Total Cheats: 2.5 (2 if you used the chia seeds)

DINNER: Cheat-Free Stir-Fry with shrimp or grass-fed steak
Total Cheats: 2—from the meat and oil

Cheats: You've only used 4.5 Cheats (or 4 if you had the chia). You have 3.5 remaining.

Day 5

BREAKFAST: Anti-inflammatory Shake; bowl of fresh berries; 1 cup of black coffee
Total Cheats: 0

LUNCH: The Basalt; simple salad of mixed greens with Magic Lime Dressing
Total Cheats: 2.5 from the bacon and salmon

DINNER: Favorite Roast Chicken OR Philly Cheesesteak Soup; large salad with French Dijon dressing; with Cheat Confetti Parmesan Crisps
Total Cheats: 3—from the meat, oil, and cheese

Cheats: You've used 5.5 Cheats. You have 2.5 remaining.

Day 6

BREAKFAST: Eggs Benedict: 2 poached eggs with 1 slice of Canadian bacon and ⅓ pound of sautéed spinach
Total Cheats: 0 (first protein, fat is free!)

LUNCH: Za'atar Grilled Chicken Strips with Warm Applewood Bacon Soup or Di's Lentil Soup
Total Cheats: 1.5—from the chicken and oil

DINNER: Slow-Cooker Fire-Roasted Tomato Beef Chili (2 servings); 1 pound broccoli with Cheat Confetti Parmesan Crisps
Total Cheats: 5—if you eat the full pound, only 4 cheats

Cheats: You've used 6.5 Cheats (5.5 if you ate the full pound of broccoli). You have 1.5 remaining.

Day 7

Breakfast: Orange Creamsicle Shake
Total Cheats: 0!

Lunch: The Famous Puréed PEERtrainer Energy Soup OR Weight-Loss Shortcut Soup OR Carrot Ginger Soup; Brian's Sweet Potato and Coconut Meatballs
Total Cheats: 3—from the coconut, coconut milk, and meat

Dinner: Tequila Lime Chicken with black beans (2 Cheats); Simple Sautéed Spinach
Total Cheats: 2—from the chicken and oil

Cheats: You've used 5 Cheats. You have 3 remaining.

THE CHEAT INCENTIVES

In addition to the Cheats you can earn by eating ½ pound of greens after 5 P.M. or by eating chia and flax seeds, there is one more way you can earn extra Cheats this week!

You can earn **two extra Cheats for the week** when you put an alarm in your phone that has a positive message related to your goal or a reminder of something that makes you really happy. You alarm could be a mantra (my "alarm" is "This Is the Year") or a goal such as "150 is almost here." This trick brings your mental focus back to your goal and helps keep you on track. When focus and goals are married together, we can achieve things so much more quickly. Set the alarm to go off once or even twice a day, at different times. (If for whatever reason, adding this to your phone doesn't work for you, putting it as the background or screensaver on your computer screen or writing it down and taping that note to your mirror will work, too.)

Week Two to Do

+ Be sure to weigh in if you aren't weighing in every day
+ Read your goal and see if it's changed. If so, change it!

Week Two Exercise Plan

- Do the Egoscue Exercises 5 to 8 every other day (it takes only 10 minutes!)
- Be active for 20 minutes *total* every other day. The time can be broken up however you want; you can spend 20 minutes walking, or just 5 minutes walking and 15 minutes playing Wii Tennis, or 10 minutes walking the dog twice a day. Just get in your 20 minutes.

CHAPTER 7

Cheat System Plan
Week Three

Eat the Eats, Learn to Cheat

By this point in the Cheat System, you are enjoying the Eats more than you thought you would—and have incorporated some of our soup, shake, and PEERtrainer recipes in your everyday life. It may have gotten frustrating at some point to read, over and over again, that vegetables make you feel full because you might not have felt full every time you ate. You might still want a pound of cheese or bacon with your breakfast.

But you have been eating the Cheat System way for only two weeks and sometimes your body takes time to adjust. We've noticed that all of our PEERtrainer members who try the Cheat System way of eating experience a transition period, and you're still in the beginning.

There will be a moment—and if it hasn't happened yet, it will soon—where you are open to trying everything in the produce aisle because you've begun to draw connections between how fresh food like salad and processed foods like pizza affect how your body feels. Your body starts to link the good feeling to healthy foods and the bad feeling to unhealthy foods, so the choice is easy. You will be shocked when you crave a salad and pass up the pizza.

You also have noticed that your taste buds are starting to change. You may be noticing that foods taste sweeter or richer or that your palate can detect any hint of sugar or sweetness. (If you chose a rich dessert as a Cheat, you definitely know what I mean!) This is natural; the change happens nearly every time people try the Cheat System.

Eating the Cheat System way will also help you figure out what Cheats are worth it for you and which foods you don't want to waste Cheats on. For me, it's easy to pass up bread so I can have bacon. In addition to realizing what Cheats you really love, you'll begin to notice which foods you may have been binging on that stopped you from losing weight before on other diets you've tried.

Perhaps you've fallen off the wagon and ended up gorging on Girl Scout cookies one night or splurged and had a margarita that turned into four with your friends. In those instances, it's really important to remember not to be hard on yourself. Don't beat yourself up over a Girl Scout cookie.

Because the second you start beating yourself up, you'll go backwards. The Cheat System is designed to help you get over those little bumps in the road without turning into the type of person we all were at some point. The person who read everything about how to lose weight but didn't take any action. The person who decided to go on a diet but gave up because it was too overwhelming. The person who has a fridge full of produce but ends up ordering take-out.

So if you tussled with a package of Thin Mints, you shouldn't worry! Pick yourself up, dust yourself off, and get back to eating your Eats. You haven't failed, you haven't lost, and you're definitely still in the game. Get back to eating your eats—and if you want a Girl Scout cookie for one of your Cheats, have one!

In Week Three of the Cheat System, I'd like you to go to **six Cheats.** Week Three offers a few incentives to earn another Cheat for the week—by adding **garlic, cinnamon, ginger, or turmeric in at least one meal.**

If this sounds intimidating, you don't have to do it! But if you want to earn that Cheat, adding spices into meals is a relatively easy thing to do and can transform the taste of a meal from bland to delicious. Grocery stores sell peeled garlic cloves and even jars of pre-minced garlic for you to use.

Cinnamon is easy to add to shakes and soups; using ginger is an easy way to flavor stir-fries, and it's surprisingly delicious on fish like salmon. Tumeric is used in a lot of cuisines. I put ginger in my tea. I sprinkle cinnamon on my sweet potato.

Some of the recipes in this week's meal plan include ginger, turmeric, and cinnamon, but really if you are adventurous, the possibilities are endless. The rules from last week still applies: you can still earn an extra Cheat for eating a ½ pound of greens after 5 p.m., or half a Cheat by eating chia or flax. But you can still only earn two extra Cheats each day, even if you add a spice to your meals every night this week, chia seeds, and eat pounds of greens.

CHEAT WEEK THREE MEAL PLAN

+ Eat your Eats. You have 6 Cheats per day.
+ Take your fish oil capsules every day.
+ You can earn one extra Cheat for eating ½ pound of greens after 5 p.m.
+ You can earn an extra ½ Cheat this week for eating a serving of chia or flax seeds.
+ You can earn an extra ½ Cheat if you add cinnamon, ginger, or turmeric in one of your meals each day.

Week Three Meal Plan

Day 1

Breakfast: ½ cup of steel cut oatmeal (1.5 Cheats) with 1 large chicken sausage link (1.5 Cheats) mixed with mushrooms, onions, and sautéed spinach (eggless omelet!)
Total Cheats: 1.5—from the oats (first protein is free)

Lunch: Creamy Chicken Salad (1.5 Cheats) atop power greens (mix of kale, mustard greens, and mixed greens)
Total Cheats: 1.5—from the chicken and yogurt

DINNER: Night Eater's Best Friend Salad (2.5 Cheats); 6 almonds (0.5 Cheats); 1 cup of tea
Total Cheats: 2.5 (first healthy fat is free!)

Cheats: You've used 5.5 Cheats. You have 5.5 remaining.

Day 2

BREAKFAST: Chocolate Decadence Shake
Total Cheats: 0 (first shake is free!)

LUNCH: Carrot Ginger Soup OR Butternut Squash Soup with Za'atar Grilled Chicken Strips or whatever spice you like!
Total Cheats: 2.5—from the coconut milk, oil, and chicken

SNACK: 1 apple
Total Cheats: 0 (first fruit free!)

DINNER: ¼ pound grass-fed steak (1.5 Cheats); 1 sweet potato; large green salad with simple French Dijon dressing or roasted asparagus (1 Cheat); one 4-ounce glass of chardonnay or Argentinian cabernet (1 Cheat)
Total Cheats: 3.5 (from the steak and the wine)

Cheats: You've used 6 Cheats. You have 0 remaining.

Day 3

BREAKFAST: Chocolate Almond Sea Salt Shake; 1 cup of coffee
Total Cheats: 0 (first shake is free!)

LUNCH: Cheat-Free Stir-Fry with salmon
Total Cheats: 2.5 from the oil and the salmon

DINNER: Chicken with Peruvian Green Sauce (2.5); Cauliflower Rice (.5); 1 pound of sauteed spinach (you've earned a Cheat!); one 4-ounce glass of wine (1)
Total Cheats: 4 (3 if you eat the spinach)

Cheats: You've used 6.5 Cheats here, 5.5 if you ate the spinach.

Day 4

BREAKFAST: South of the Border Eggs OR 2 scrambled eggs with leftover spinach
Total Cheats: 0! (first protein, fat is free!)

LUNCH: Butternut Squash Soup OR Weight-Loss Shortcut Soup (1 Cheat); 1 serving of Easy Italian Herb Baked Turkey (1.5 Cheats)
Total Cheats: 2.5—from the oil, the coconut milk, and the turkey

SNACK: Apple with 1 tablespoon of almond butter (1 Cheat)
Total Cheats: 1

DINNER: Japanese Chili Salmon (2 Cheats); leftover Cheat-Free Stir-Fry; cucumber-tomato salad (0); large piping hot cup of herbal tea
Total Cheats: 2—from the salmon, oil, and avocado

Cheats: You've used 5.5 cheats. You have .5 remaining.

Day 5

BREAKFAST: Chocolate Raspberry Torte Shake
Total Cheats: 0 (first shake is free!)

LUNCH: The Famous Puréed PEERtrainer Energy Soup with leftover Japanese Chili Salmon
Total Cheats: 3—from the coconut milk, salmon, and oil

DINNER: Ginger Salmon with Bok Choy and Spinach
Total Cheats: 2

Cheats: You've had 5 cheats! You have 1 remaining Cheat!

Day 6

BREAKFAST: Chocolate Almond Sea Salt Shake
Total Cheats: 0 (first shake is free!)

Lunch: Slow-Cooker Chicken and Spinach Soup; sweet potato (2 Cheats) OR 2 servings of soup with a serving of chicken OR 2 pieces of salmon sashimi and a large mixed-green salad with hot green tea
Total Cheats: 2

Eating out: Chipotle Bowl (chicken), ½ serving of beans, lettuce, salsa, golf-sized portion of avocado
Total Cheats: 3

Dinner: PEERtrainer Bacon Avocado Burgers (3 Cheats); ½ pound of broccoli; Simple Sautéed Spinach; piña colada (1 Cheat) OR one 4-ounce glass of wine
Total Cheats: 3—from the meat, bacon, avocado, coconut milk, and pineapple juice or wine. You earned 1 Cheat from the greens!

Cheats: You've used 6 Cheats (if you ate out for lunch, 5 Cheats if you did not). You have 0 left (1 left if you did not eat out).

Day 7

Breakfast: Power Workout Breakfast OR Carrot Cake Smoothie OR two hard-boiled eggs with leftover vegetables
Total Cheats: 0 Cheats! (first protein or shake is free!)

Lunch: Mediterranean Gourmet Power Bowl with optionals (1 Cheat)
Total Cheats: 1—from the oil and goat cheese

Dinner: ¼-pound grass-fed steak OR fish with Orange Ginger Sauce and salad with ⅓ of avocado (2.5 Cheats) OR Mint and Shallot Halibut with Kale and Oven-Roasted Tomatoes (1.5 Cheats), salad with ⅓ avocado (1 Cheat)
Total Cheats: 2.5—from the steak or halibut, avocado, and oil

Cheats: You've had 3.5 Cheats. You have 2.5 left.

THE CHEAT INCENTIVES

There is one more way you can earn two extra Cheats this week!

You can earn **two extra Cheats for the week** if you send yourself an e-mail in the evening, every day this week, detailing everything you're appreciative of. The e-mail should have the subject line of tomorrow's date and you should send it in the evening so you can read it the following morning.

List everything you're excited about or grateful for. It can be the smallest thing, like finding hairbands for a dollar, to big important things like being thankful that your partner or parents are in good health. The list should include anything you're personally psyched about—not everything on the list has to be profound or life-changing. I've literally included, "I'm so psyched about adding a third blanket to my bed because I'm finally warm at night!" to my e-mails. If you send an e-mail to yourself every night this week, you will earn two extra Cheats.

Week Three to Do

+ Hurray! You've through the three weeks. Record your weight, review your goal, and keep going.

Week Three Exercise Plan

+ Do the Egoscue Exercises 9 to 12 every other day (it only takes 10 minutes!)
+ Be active for 20 minutes *total* every other day. The time can be broken up however you want; you can spend 20 minutes walking, or just 5 minutes walking and 15 minutes playing Wii Tennis, or 10 minutes walking the dog twice a day. Just get in your 20 minutes.

CHAPTER 8

Your Magic Fridge

"It's impossible," said pride. "It's risky," said experience.
"It's pointless," said reason. "Give it a try," whispered the heart.

—UNKNOWN

I want to start this chapter by saying that reading this chapter is entirely optional. I've discovered, as the leader at PEERtrainer, that some people find "prepping" for a new way of eating helpful while others hate the process and just want to start the program already!

The Magic Fridge is the biggest shortcut there is to eating the Cheat System way. It will tell you not only what to get rid of from your refrigerator and cupboards but also what you should buy at the grocery store, from spices that help the Eats taste great to the Eats themselves so you reduce the chances of finding yourself staring into the fridge wondering what you're going to eat for breakfast, lunch, or dinner.

The Magic Fridge was developed at the request of PEERtrainer members who loved the Cheat Sheet but wanted to go one step further and just have a shopping list for everything they would need to be successful on our plan. From the kitchen tools that will save you time and energy to foods that you can buy at any time, freeze, and eat later, the advice I give you in this chapter has helped set many people up for success eating the Cheat System way.

The Magic Fridge does *not* include recipes for low-fat cheesecake or whole wheat pizza. The reasons why should be obvious: first, we don't advocate for fake "healthy" foods on Cheat System. We concentrate on meals made with whole, natural, actually healthy foods. The Magic Fridge focuses on the foods that should make up 80 percent of your plate at every meal—the Eats that give you the high nutrients necessary for sustainable and hunger-free weight loss.

I'll be honest. I would still rather pick up a slice of pizza any day of the week than cook a Cheat-free meal. A slice of pizza is fast, tastes great, and is really easy—but unfortunately, now that I'm over forty, I can't control my portions anymore. One slice of pizza leaves me hungry and I end up gorging on almost the whole pie. The solution is creating high-nutrient meals that taste great, which don't require slaving in the kitchen all day—and that's what the Magic Fridge will give you.

For those of you who love food and love to cook, you're going to love what the Magic Fridge does for you—it's basically a sous-chef in the form of a chapter. The fact is, if I had to choose between working all day in the kitchen to make a delicious meal or eating bland food, I wouldn't have been able to sustain my weight loss of over sixty pounds. But with the Magic Fridge, you don't have to make that choice. It helps you create truly delicious low-Cheat or even Cheat-free meals without being in the kitchen all day. (However, if you want to spend time making a meal or soup in bulk so you have food prepared for the week, we'll show you how to do that, too.)

Now, when I take the time to cook I know that it's an investment. What do I mean by saying it's an investment? Here's how I like to think of it: **If I spend time making food, it will be the gift that keeps on giving. I may spend forty-five minutes making something that tastes great, but I'll see the results on the scale. And if I make extra, I won't have to cook later today, tomorrow, or later this week!**

I'll make a staple, like grilled chicken or the greens tapenade, which will last me for a few days in the fridge so I can grab it any time I want to make a salad. If I make a soup, I'll make a lot of it so it lasts a few days or can be put in the freezer for later consumption.

When I first mentioned the concept of a constant resource of good, nutrient-rich food to my husband, he remarked that it reminded him of "The Magic Pot," an Indonesian story he heard as a child, about a rice bowl that was always filled with food. That's why I decided to name this chapter "Your Magic Fridge" because that's what it's going to feel like: a fridge filled with food.

You can go to the grocery store and start this today. Think of it as a fun adventure where you're replacing the old with the new.

There are four easy steps to the Magic Fridge:

1. Clean out what's not working for you.
2. Buy essential kitchen tools.
3. Fill your fridge with must-have foods.
4. Take spice shortcuts.

CLEAN OUT WHAT'S NOT WORKING FOR YOU

The number one thing I tell PEERtrainer members and people interested in weight loss to do is to clean out their cupboards and their fridge. The rule of thumb is to clear out anything that you know is bad for you and takes five minutes or less to prepare and eat. When you're starving, you're going to turn to those foods if they are available in the cupboard or in the fridge for you to eat. By removing the foods you *know* are bad for you, you eliminate that option.

Willpower goes out the window when you're face-to-face with a bag of potato chips. Be honest with yourself and get rid of anything that falls into the category of a food that's easy, tasty, and a Cheat. I already hear what you're thinking: "There's no way my husband/ wife/boyfriend/girlfriend/son/daughter/kids/roommate is going to let me do that." My husband used to regularly bring home an Entenmann's cake from the store. I asked him not to—I couldn't resist them!—and he replied, "You obviously don't know men and hunger." He refused to stop. (He also used to bring home pints of ice cream, but for some reason, that wasn't a problem for me. Ice cream just wasn't a trigger food, but that cake in the fridge was.) I knew that the moment I had a bad day, I was going straight to that cake. It took two years for him to listen, but he finally did and stopped bringing home the cake. Don't give up asking for what you need. And after your roommate/boyfriend/girlfriend/wife/husband/kids eat the delicious foods you prepare as part of your diet, they might be tempted to give up whatever food is tempting you and try the Cheat System way, too! You never know. . . .

BUY ESSENTIAL KITCHEN TOOLS

The second step is to make your life easier by buying a few key kitchen tools. You may already have some of these in your kitchen! (Note that I assume that you already own a saucepan, a casserole dish, and other true basics.) There's no need to go "fancy" and buy luxury brands. Just shoot for something that has great reviews online or is a trusted brand, like OXO, Cuisinart, Calphalon, and others.

The Five Essential Kitchen Tools

1. A stick immersion blender

It's relatively inexpensive and is key to making healthy soups and purées. Don't try to use your existing food blender; it's not the same. The engine of a typical blender can be easily overwhelmed and burn out puréeing vegetables and greens. An immersion blender enables you to make greens like spinach and kale taste delicious by pulverizing them and bringing out their nutrients. Once the greens are pulverized, you can mix them with whatever base or taste you want, like salsa or guacamole. Typically priced around twenty-five dollars, an immersion blender is a wise investment, especially if you like soups, sauces, and shakes.

2. A rice cooker . . . for so much more than rice

You'll find that this is an incredible time saving tool. You put your food in, walk away, and come back to it completely ready. Quinoa and vegetables can be made in a rice cooker fast, and there's no need to even turn the stove on!

3. Freezer-safe containers

These are a lifesaver when you choose to cook in bulk. You can use them to freeze soups, stocks, sauces, and traditional proteins. Buy a couple in a variety of sizes to try at first, and later you can buy more in the sizes you use most often, if needed.

4. A great knife and a cutting board

Okay, so technically these are two tools, but they work hand in hand. Cutting vegetables will be much, much easier with a good knife than with a substandard one. Buying a cutting board that is strong and durable will make a difference, too. If you don't like what you have now, this is a good excuse to buy replacements.

5. Two large salad bowls

Many salad bowls are smaller than they should be, and that's because people think salads should be a side dish. On Cheat System, they are definitely not side dishes! Buying two large salad bowls will help you mix up a salad quickly and easily. And buying two makes it more likely that you'll have one clean when you want to make a salad! Try to find one that can hold about 8 to 10 cups of food—so you'll have room to include not just greens but veggies, a protein, and your dressing without making a mess. If you already have a large mixing bowl, don't be afraid to use that—it's the same thing in different packaging.

Other handy kitchen tools can include a good slotted spoon, which is great for sautéing kale and other greens; a large stockpot, which allows you to make soups in bulk and store the rest directly in the fridge; and a water pitcher, which has been shown to increase the amount of water you'll drink during the day more than just relying on filling up your glass from the tap or using bottled water. Also, if you have a pitcher of water, it's super easy to flavor the entire pitcher with cucumber, lemons, or limes, just like they do at the best spas.

FILL YOUR FRIDGE WITH MUST-HAVE FOODS

I want you to have at least two go-to foods in your fridge at all times. These are Eats that you *love*, which you can literally pull out and eat on the spot. Having these in your fridge is an insurance policy for when you feel like "you're so hungry you could eat a house." These should be healthy, energy-filled snacks that are easy to prepare, foods you don't have to think about too much to create a meal out of. Some of my favorites include hummus, cucumbers, tabouli, quinoa with mixed greens, avocado squeezed with lemon, and sliced tomato and cucumber salad, beans, sweet potatoes, chicken breasts, chili, hard-boiled eggs, and soups. Soups (see pages 189 to 194 for our PEER-trainer soup recipes) are always at the top of my list. They are the ultimate Magic Fridge staple.

The list goes on and on and can be anything you want, provided your go-to foods are Eats. Having these on hand will help you make the right choices when you're starving and want food *now*.

There are three different kinds of foods that I want you to get used to having in the house and buying every single time you're in the grocery store.

The Three Must-Have Foods in Every Magic Fridge

1. Frozen vegetables

This can be whatever you like, but I want you to have some vegetables—especially some greens like spinach and kale—that only take a few minutes in the microwave to prepare whenever you're hungry.

At all times, have at least two 1-pound bags of frozen spinach or collard greens or kale in your freezer. Organic is around two dollars per bag and the nutrient content doesn't change from frozen to fresh or organic to non-organic. Yes, buying organic is preferable, but if that's too expensive for you, non-organic frozen greens are fine. Buy frozen greens and you'll always have something on hand to up the nutrient content of everything you eat.

2. Huge containers of fresh greens, spring greens, and spinach

You can literally throw these into every meal you make on Cheat System, so every meal that you eat has more nutritional "heft." I like to have fresh, prewashed salad mixes and greens in my fridge because I'll add some to every meal I make. If you can do fresh, do fresh!

You can stick fresh spinach leaves in any smoothie you make because it's completely masked by the other flavors in the smoothie. (I do this when I make smoothies for my kids.) You can throw fresh spinach in rice, beans, wraps, dips, underneath a main dish like salmon or chicken, even in omelets. It's really versatile and often the flavor of spinach "disappears" when you have stronger flavors mixed in. Try it!

3. Condiments for the spice shortcuts

You probably have condiments in your fridge now like ketchup, mayonnaise, and soy sauce—which often have added ingredients and tons of sugar and fat. You can replace the flavors of those condiments with the ingredients for the spice shortcuts I'm going to share with you.

But in terms of a shopping list for the condiments that make up the spice shortcuts, you should buy and have on hand the following: garlic, fresh limes and lemons, mustard, red pepper flakes, olive oil, cumin, turmeric, Adobo (a spice blend made by Goya), avocados, cilantro, ginger, wasabi, oregano, basil, thyme, and coconut milk. It's okay if some of these are in dried form, though fresh is usually a little bit more flavorful. But do what you are able to do!

TAKE SPICE SHORTCUTS

One of the best ways to lose weight and love your food is to discover what flavors and spices you love. What is it that you love about the taste of pasta meat sauce? To replicate the flavor of a tasty Italian sausage sauce you can use tomatoes with basil, thyme, oregano, bay leaves, and red pepper flakes in a recipe for a healthy tomato soup that tastes like the sauce you love.

It's really easy to use spices to create delicious meals that taste similar to those bad-for-you "Cheat" foods. And once you start to use the spice shortcuts listed here, you will develop a sense of what works together to make meals taste great. Feel free to experiment with your spice rack and your must-have condiments!

These spice combos make anything taste great!

- **Fresh lime, cilantro, and red pepper flakes** for Mexican-inspired meats, fish, soups, and vegetables
- **Lemon, olive oil, and fresh garlic** for Mediterranean-style fish or salads
- **Mustard, olive oil, and lemon** for grilled vegetables, salads and chicken; you can give this a little kick by using spicy mustard instead of yellow
- **Cilantro, avocado, and lemon purée,** which adds a crisp flair to vegetables and salads
- **Cumin, turmeric, and ginger** for a Middle Eastern, Indian-inspired mix to chicken, beans, and meat
- **Curry powder or Muchi Curry** (available at Whole Foods) for Asian Indian flavors
- **Ginger, garlic, and red onion,** which is great for all meats (it's the base used for chicken tikka)
- **Oregano, basil, and thyme** for Italian-inspired meals (great for vegetables, chicken, and fish)
- **Wasabi, lemon, and ginger** for Japanese-inspired fish and vegetables like asparagus and broccoli
- **Coconut milk, red pepper flakes, lime, and onions** for Thai-inspired dishes, and great for meats, vegetables, and fish

You can also use these spices to make easy salad dressings. The Magic Lime Dressing (page 202), which I think is quite delicious and incredibly versatile, only has three ingredients: the juice of two limes, a pinch of salt, and four shakes of red pepper flakes. Though you can add ¼ of an avocado or some olive oil to it, that's not necessary to make a delicious dressing for any salad (or as a sauce to top protein like chicken or fish).

Remember, the most important thing is that you learn what you like and you understand how not only to make great-tasting, nutrient-rich foods when you are at home cooking but also how to find those same meals out and about in your day. If you find that you like tomatoes and onions and avocado, you will start to look for those combinations at restaurants and you will find them.

"Your Magic Fridge" teaches you the basics of the Cheat System and it will create the good habits that will make you successful over the next three weeks. You'll start to see yourself eat better because it's easy to do when these foods are in your fridge; you'll feel more full because you're eating nutrient-rich foods, and you'll take small steps to make vegetables taste better than you ever imagined, discovering flavors that you never thought you'd like—and that you'll soon love.

PART THREE

Cheaters for Life

CHAPTER 9

The Cheating Gourmet

How to Create a Magic Kitchen (with More Than 100 Recipes for Cheating and Eating!)

It's not the critic who counts . . . [it's] the man who is actually in the arena.

—TEDDY ROOSEVELT

Almost a year ago, my mother-in-law—who is a brilliant, incredible chef—went to our local Indian store and bought over twenty-five common Indian spices to put in our cupboard. After she left, I put those spices away in a cupboard, and I am not kidding when I say that I was *afraid* of that cupboard! For six months. I didn't know the first thing to do with cardamom, turmeric, or black mustard seeds—and I really didn't want to. I knew there were lots of very healthy Indian dishes that my husband loved. But cooking seemed like so much time and effort even with spices I knew. Using spices I wasn't even remotely familiar with was way too intimidating for me.

Eventually, my mother-in-law came over again and showed me how to make her delicious fish curry. She took me through every single step, and of course, since she was there, it turned out perfectly. But something else happened that day—I was no longer afraid of the cupboard. A few weeks later, once I had become confident in being able to make the curry, she showed me how to make another recipe. Now, a few years later, I know how to make three or four of my husband's favorite dishes—and trying a new Indian dish doesn't intimidate me anymore.

If you're the kind of person who gets nervous about using cookbooks and online recipe databases, or has no idea how your friends are able to make what they serve at dinner parties, you are not alone. If you are afraid to ask what the different herbs are in the produce section of your grocery store, you're not alone. Grocery stores can incredibly overwhelming—especially a place like Whole Foods that has *so much stuff*. I'm still intimidated by leeks; I actually don't even know what one would look like in a store! And even though a few friends of mine have explained how to prepare and cook leeks, I'm still nervous. I really love potato leek soup when I dine out, but will I ever make it for myself? Probably not—and that's okay.

If you have no idea how to make hard-boiled eggs, to prepare beans that aren't in a can, or to cook in a slow cooker, you're definitely not alone. And if you're interested in learning, we're now going to teach you all those techniques. Everything you need to know to successfully Cheat and Eat—whether you want to cook, or want to avoid it like the plague—is in this chapter.

If you are at an advanced level—and love to spend time making new, healthy dishes—this chapter is for you, too. We've included advanced techniques and we teach you how to become a "cheating gourmet." Whatever your level, we have it here.

YOUR MAGIC KITCHEN

I'm not going to assume you know anything about preparing or cooking food in this chapter. (So if you fancy yourself an amateur chef, you'll probably know a lot of the basics I'm going to share.) A lot of us—including myself—haven't spent days in our mom's kitchen or hours on the couch watching Food Network learning how to make the perfect marinade or how to poach an egg. If you're that person, you're going to love the Magic Kitchen.

No One Is Perfect

You don't have to cook perfectly; in fact, most professional chefs would tell you that imperfect cooking typically ends up tastier than someone who follows a recipe or cookbook to the letter.

If you don't have an ingredient, go without it. If you don't have the right pan, feel free to use something similar. After all, an omelet that falls apart is just a scramble: it has the same ingredients, the same taste, and the same number of Cheats. Don't beat yourself up over a scrambled egg. Don't make perfect the enemy of the good.

Cheatify, Cheatify, Cheatify!

The recipes in this chapter are designed for Cheating and Eating. However, if one of your favorite meals is not adapted in this chapter, you can always *cheatify* it. Think of Joel Fuhrman's term: G-BOMBS: Greens, Beans, Onions, Mushrooms, Berries, Seeds and Nuts. These are the best-bang-for-your-buck nutrients. Any time you add onions, greens, cooked mushrooms, beans, vegetables, seeds, nuts, or berries to a recipe, you are successfully cheatifying that recipe. Think of the balancing scale: by adding those healthy Eats, you're tipping the whole meal in that direction. You'll notice we have cheatified a lot of common dishes in our recipes. For example, we cheatified BLTs (The Basalt, page 211), ranch dressing (Spicy Ranch Dressing, page 282), and even margaritas (Muscle Recovery Margaritas, page 294).

You can also do this when you're eating out. For example, recently our collaborator on this book went out to a Japanese ramen noodle restaurant. She ordered what seemed to be the healthiest option—the vegetable ramen soup, which had a vegetable broth, spinach noodles, chicken instead of pork, and lots of veggies—but the menu had an option to add kale and cabbage, so she did that, asking for double portions of each. Instant cheatify!

THE BASICS

A lot of us have no idea how to make rice from scratch, how to make greens taste great, or even what quinoa is. In this section, we'll go over a few basics that you might not find in the recipes themselves.

Cooking with (Less) Oil

A great way to use less oil when cooking is to let the pan properly heat first *before* adding it. Put the pan on the stove and let it heat up. After a few minutes, test the pan's temperature by taking a drop of water and flicking it to the pan. If the water sizzles and evaporates, your pan is hot enough. (If not, wait another minute and try again.)

This will not only allow you to use less oil, but will also prevent food from sticking to the pan. There's a lot less cleanup—and a lot fewer calories.

"WHICH OIL SHOULD I USE?"

For most of our Cheat System recipes, we advocate using olive oil or coconut oil. You might have heard that olive oil is toxic when heated—and while that is true, it only applies when you heat olive oil past its specific "smoke point."

Every oil has its own smoke point, which differs depending on how it's made and processed. As long as you don't heat the oil above that temperature, nothing bad will happen to you or your food. Here are the smoke points for the oils we recommend on Cheat System:

> Extra-virgin olive oil: 375 degrees F
> Virgin olive oil: 391 degrees F
> Unrefined coconut oil: 350 degrees F
> Refined coconut oil: 450 degrees F

Most of these oils won't approach their smoke points if you only heat your stove to medium (which is usually the case for most of our recipes). However, if you're going to cook something in the oven at high temperature—for example, if you are roasting vegetables or making sweet potato fries—you are better off using an oil with a high smoke point, such as refined coconut oil.

When buying oil, the cheapest olive oil you can buy is usually best. By "cheap" I mean the oil with the simplest processing. If you find a company with oil you like, buying their "virgin" or "pomace" (which is one step down from extra virgin and has a smoke point of 460 degrees) will be fine.

However, when you're making a recipe where the taste of the olive oil will really matter, adding some great or even flavored extra-virgin olive oil is ideal. Having garlic-infused extra-virgin olive oil on hand to add to sautéed vegetables or to use in a salad dressing can add an extra dash of delicious.

How to Boil Eggs

Hard-boiled eggs are great to have on hand while Cheating and Eating. It's a quick protein when you're in a rush, is incredibly versatile (you can eat it on a salad, as part of a salad topping, or by itself), and can be a great alternative to hot eggs.

Making hard-boiled eggs isn't difficult. First, put the eggs in a pot. Cover the eggs completely, with at least an inch of water over the entire egg(s). Bring the water to a boil. As soon as the water starts to boil, reduce the heat to low and simmer for 10 to 12 minutes. Prepare another bowl with ice water. Remove the eggs with a slotted spoon and put them into the ice water carefully. Once the eggs are cooled, drain the water and store the eggs in a covered container in the refrigerator. Hard-boiled eggs last about five days in the refrigerator.

How to Make Greens Taste Great

Sautéed kale, spinach, Swiss chard, mustard greens—virtually any leafy green—can taste great. The trick is to prepare it correctly. To start, heat a skillet (frying pan) or saucepan (what you'd cook pasta sauce in) over medium to high heat. Add a little bit of oil, then add chopped greens. (If you like garlic, you can add minced garlic before you add in the greens.) Add a half cup of water, cover, and lower heat to medium.

After a few minutes, check on the greens to see if the water has evaporated; if it has, add a little more. Stir the greens around in the pan, so it cooks evenly. Depending on which green you're cooking and in what quantity, it will take five to fifteen minutes to properly sauté your greens. If you're in doubt, try it out!

How to Make Quinoa

A lot of us are intimidated by quinoa. Perhaps it's because the word is confusing to say (it's pronounced *keen-wah*), and when you look at it in its dry form, quinoa looks a lot like birdseed—which is no wonder because it is actually a seed. It's nutty and really satisfying. It's more nutritious and easier to make than traditional rice—and can be substituted for rice in nearly any recipe.

One cup of dry quinoa makes 3 cups of quinoa. You have to rinse quinoa first, to remove its saponins (a substance that naturally occurs on the outside of the quinoa grains to deter insects and birds). Rinse the quinoa by either using a strainer (with thin holes) or by running fresh water over the quinoa in a pot and draining it.

Place 1 cup of quinoa and 2 cups water in a medium saucepan on medium to high heat, and bring it to a boil. Once it's boiling, reduce the heat and simmer for ten to fifteen minutes, until all the water has evaporated. You'll be able to tell that the quinoa is done when its grains are translucent and its outer layer has separated.

How to Make Beans

Up until very recently, I was totally okay using premade beans in cans. I knew about BPA and that I shouldn't use cans, but I did anyway. It's not like I was eating Velveeta! But once I learned how easy it was to make beans in bulk from scratch, I started doing that and rarely go back (though I do always keep beans in a can in my cupboard so I have some just in case). Beans you prepare yourself taste better than what comes in a can, and though it takes time, I feel like making beans is totally worth it.

In order to cook beans from scratch, you need to soak them first.

(Lentils, split peas, and black-eyed peas don't need to be soaked.) Pick through the beans and discard any discolored or shriveled beans from the bag. Rinse the beans well and then put them in a stockpot. Cover the beans with water. If you are making a one-pound bag (2 cups dried beans), you will get 6 cups of cooked beans at the end. Cover the pan and refrigerate it overnight.

The next day, drain the soaked beans. Cover the beans with water and add any herbs or spices you want (avoid salt). Bring the beans and water to a boil, then simmer gently, uncovered, stirring occasionally until beans are tender. (The time depends on the type of bean you're making, but it usually takes about forty-five minutes to an hour.) Add more water if the beans are not completely covered at any point in the process. You can also toss beans and water in a slow cooker—it's super easy and you don't have to watch at all! Beans can also be made in a pressure cooker and can save you tons of time.

When beans are tender, drain and use as you want. (If you're going to reserve some for later, immerse the beans in cold water until they are cool, then drain. You can freeze prepared beans in 1- to 2-cup packages.) This might sound like a lot of work, but I promise if you eat beans regularly, it's worth it!

Cheat Confetti

"Sprinkling" Cheats throughout your meals is the number one reason PEERtrainer members find eating the Cheat System way to be so doable—and delicious.

 "If I have caramelized walnuts on my salad as Cheat Confetti, I'm digging until the very bottom of the bowl so I can make sure I eat every single last one!"
—Erin, Florida

Throughout this chapter, you'll find a bunch of ideas for Cheat Confetti including Parmesan crisps, bacon bits, power green confetti, goat cheese, potato chips, Cheat sausage confetti, caramelized walnuts, cinnamon baked almonds, goat cheese polenta squares, even crumbled French fries! This is an abbreviated list but I know that you'll find your perfect Cheat Confetti. Maybe it will be adding French fries confetti to your steak salad, or adding bacon to anything.

Adding some Cheat Confetti—a topping to the party, not making it the main meal—is a great way to make a salad, a soup, or an entrée taste delicious without going overboard or wasting a day's worth of Cheats.

Don't have large amounts of Cheat Confetti in the fridge if you can't stay away from it. Make only individualized servings if you think it's a potential trigger food.

THE RECIPES

With the help of our members at PEERtrainer, we've included **more than 100 recipes** for cheating and eating in this chapter!

Eat Any Recipe, Any Time

Though we separated our recipes into categories by what people typically eat, feel free to use any recipe for each of the three meals every day on Cheat System. Personally, I love having Jackie's Vail Chophouse Salad (mine, adapted from the Vail Chophouse) (page 199) or the Savory Rosemary Chicken Salad with Cheat Confetti Parmesan Crisps (pages 206 and 210) in the morning as breakfast, though I completely understand that most people have an image of what breakfast is in their head and a salad is not for breakfast. That's totally okay.

When I lived abroad, I noticed that the locals ate "weird" things for breakfast like schnitzel or cucumber, tomato and onion salad. Once I tried it, I realized why: these foods provided more energy than what I was used to eating for breakfast. And that's important because we do a lot after breakfast: we get ourselves ready for the day, get our families ready for the day, and use our brain and body to do what we need to.

In many cultures, the biggest meal of the day is lunch. And after

I had eaten that way for a while, it made sense to me. You've been going, going, going all morning; then you eat lunch, and what do you do? You keep going, going, going.

One of the reasons Americans eat a huge dinner is because we used to be a hardworking, agricultural-based society. We worked hard physically all day. But today, for most of us that's not the case. After dinner we relax, we wind down (hopefully), we watch a little TV or read a book. We don't need a huge amount of calories to *do* anything. We're not going, going, going at night the way we are during the day. Usually, we're going to go to bed in a few hours and rest.

So, if you can somehow trick your brain into eating dinner for breakfast, or even eating dinner for lunch, do it. If you can eat salmon and vegetables in the morning like people do in Japan (where people have been shown to live the longest and healthiest), do it.

But if you can't, you're in good company; 95 percent of our members on PEERtrainer feel the same way you do. Most people simply can't stomach the thought of eating dinner for breakfast. So we've also included some traditional breakfast recipes, along with recipes for PEERtrainer shakes. The shakes are a great meal, especially when you're pressed for time (which most of us are in the morning).

Count Your Cheats!

To help you out, we've also included the number of Cheats for each recipe. Keep in mind that the Cheats listed are for *each individual serving*. For example, the Insane Man Hunger Chili recipe contains twelve servings. Each serving has two Cheats.

We've also highlighted what the Cheats *are* in each recipe, so that you can not only count your Cheats when you cook at home, but also learn what Cheats look like when you're eating out. (Also, when you know what the Cheats are in a recipe, you can easily leave those ingredients out to make the meal Cheat-free.) In each recipe, you'll see an asterisk symbol (*) by the ingredients that are Cheats, along with an explanation of why the ingredient is a Cheat at the bottom of the recipe.

Counting by Serving . . .

However, keep in mind that the exceptions to the rule—first 4 ounces of lean protein or pea rice protein, the first tablespoon of a "good" fat for the day (or if you'd like to save that for dinner), the first fruit, the first cup of coffee—are Eats and they are free, but after you had a second helping of the fat or the protein it's a Cheat—remember Eats are unlimited, at any meal! So, for example, if you see a shake has 1.5 Cheats, remember it's free if it's your first meal of the day. These recipes have Cheat numbers **without the exceptions to the rule figured in.**

The PEERtrainer Cheat System Shake is the number one weight loss kickstart that we've ever seen. So your first Cheat System Shake is Cheat free because you've earned a Cheat. The only shakes that meet this requirement are the PEERtrainer Cheat System–approved shakes. Go to http://www.peertrainer.com/cheattracker to see even more!

If You Run Out of Recipes . . .

If you try all of these recipes, there will always be new things to try on PEERtrainer.com. And we'd love to hear from you! Please send us any recipes you cheatify or share what you've done to adapt a recipe that's in the book.

BREAKFAST RECIPES & SHAKES

Anti-inflammatory Shake

Servings: 1   **Cheats/Serving: 0**

Cheat free, Cheat System–approved (after your first shake, it's 1.5).

1 scoop chocolate protein powder
1 cup frozen blueberries
1 cup unsweetened almond milk
½ pound organic spinach

Add all the ingredients to a blender and blend until smooth.

Banana Chocolate Nut Shake

Servings: 1   **Cheats/Serving: 0**

Cheat free, Cheat System–approved (after your first shake, it's 2).

1 frozen banana, chopped
½ tablespoon almond butter
8 to 10 ounces unsweetened coconut milk
1 scoop chocolate protein powder
6 ice cubes

In a blender, add the frozen banana, almond butter, and coconut milk. Blend until smooth. Add the protein powder and blend. Add the ice cubes and blend until smooth.

Brian's Mint Chocolate Chip Cookie Smoothie

Servings: 1   **Cheats/Serving: 0**

Cheat free, Cheat System–approved (after your first shake, it's 2).

The reason Brian use oats in his shakes is twofold: they're a great source of slow-digesting complex carbohydrates, which provide energy for hours, especially when combined with the protein and coconut milk in the shake; and they're naturally high in beta-glucan, a soluble fiber that promotes satiety, increases the health of our gut flora, and lowers LDL (bad) cholesterol levels. The extra carbohydrates from the oats are key for active individuals to maintain good energy levels. The cacao nibs in this recipe are a great source of antioxidants.

½ to 1 cup water
1 scoop chocolate protein powder
1 cup unsweetened coconut milk
½ scoop fiber (add more if the texture allows)
1 teaspoon cacao nibs
1 packet loose leaf mint tea, run through a coffee grinder or mixed right into the shake
¼ cup rolled oats

Add ingredients into a blender, starting with ½ cup of water. Blend, adding more water to achieve your desired thickness.

Carrot Cake Smoothie

Servings: 1   **Cheats/Serving: 0**

Cheat free, Cheat System–approved (after your first shake, it's 1.5).

Thanks to Wendy Solganik, blogger of Healthy Girl's Kitchen, for this great carrot-cake shake recipe.

1 scoop vanilla protein powder
1 cup unsweetened coconut milk
½ cup water
6 ice cubes
1 cup raw carrots
½ tablespoon chia seeds or flaxseed meal
½ scoop fiber
Dash cinnamon
Dash nutmeg
Dash ground cloves

Add all the ingredients to a blender and blend until smooth.

Chocolate Almond Sea Salt Shake

Servings: 1   **Cheats/Serving: 0**

Cheat free, Cheat System–approved (after your first shake, it's 1.5).

Inspired by Chocolove!

4 ice cubes
1 scoop chocolate protein powder
9 ounces unsweetened coconut milk
1 handful frozen organic blackberries
1 teaspoon organic vanilla extract
½ scoop fiber
1 shake sea salt

In a blender, put the ice on the bottom, and then add the other ingredients. Blend to desired consistency.

Chocolate Decadence Shake

Servings: 1   **Cheats/Serving: 0**

Cheat free, Cheat System–approved (after your first shake, it's 1.5).

A quick note: The fiber can really thicken up the smoothie—some people like that and some don't. If you are new to extra fiber in your diet, you'll want to start small and work from there.

1 scoop chocolate protein powder
1 cup unsweetened coconut milk
6 big ice cubes
½ scoop fiber
½ cup water
1 to 4 cups of greens (spinach, kale, whatever you have, fresh or frozen)
1 teaspoon unsweetened cocoa powder
1 drop vanilla extract

In a blender, mix ingredients on slow speed until blended smooth. For those with a Vitamix, try and keep it smooth by slowing the speed to avoid foaming up the mix.

Chocolate Raspberry Torte Shake

Servings: 1   **Cheats/Serving: 0**

Cheat free, Cheat System–approved (after your first shake, it's 1.5).

1 scoop chocolate protein powder
½ scoop fiber
1 cup unsweetened coconut milk or almond milk
1 cup organic raspberries
½ cup filtered water
6 ice cubes
6 nuts (optional)
Dash of cinnamon to taste (optional)

Add all the ingredients in a blender and blend until smooth.

Mango Lassi Shake

Servings: 1   **Cheats/Serving: 0**

Cheat free, Cheat System–approved (after your first shake, it's 2.5).

1 cup unsweetened almond milk or coconut milk
1 scoop vanilla protein powder
½ mango, chopped
6 ice cubes

Add all the ingredients to a blender and blend until smooth.

Orange Creamsicle Shake

Servings: 1   **Cheats/Serving: 0**

Cheat free, Cheat System–approved (after your first shake, it's 1.5).

1 cup unsweetened coconut milk
½ orange, peeled
6 ice cubes
1 scoop vanilla protein powder
½ scoop fiber
1 tablespoon chia seeds or flaxseed meal (optional)
½ cup filtered water

Combine the coconut milk, orange, and ice cubes in a blender and blend until smooth. While this is blending, add the protein powder.

Continue to run the blender while you add the fiber and chia seeds. Add water until your shake reaches the desired consistency.

Pumpkin Pie Smoothie

Servings: 1   **Cheats/Serving: 0**

Cheat free, Cheat System–approved (after your first shake, it's 1.5).

Remember, be sure when picking a protein powder to use a minimum of 20 grams of protein with no additives or dairy. Pea/rice protein or pea/potato is our recommendation. For more info, go to page 55 or go to http://www.peertrainer.com/cheatsystem to see our recommendations of protein powder.

½ cup pure pumpkin (not pumpkin pie filling)
1 scoop vanilla protein powder
½ tablespoon flaxseed meal
1 cup unsweetened coconut milk

½ scoop fiber
1 teaspoon pure vanilla extract
¼ teaspoon pumpkin pie spice
6 ice cubes

Place all ingredients into a blender and blend for 30 seconds, or until smooth.

Triple Berry Smoothie

Servings: 1   **Cheats/Serving: 0**

Cheat free, Cheat System–approved (after your first shake, it's 1.5).

1 cup frozen blueberries, raspberries, and/or blackberries
½ cup filtered water
8 ounces unsweetened coconut milk
1 scoop vanilla protein powder
1 tablespoon chia seeds (optional)
½ scoop fiber

Place the berries, water, coconut milk, protein powder, and chia seeds in a blender and blend until smooth. While continuing to blend, add the fiber supplement. Blend until smooth.

Vanilla Cinnamon Ginger Shake

Servings: 1   Cheats/Serving: 0

Cheat free, Cheat System–approved (after your first shake, it's 1.5).

1 scoop protein powder
1 cup unsweetened coconut milk
$\frac{1}{2}$ mango
$\frac{1}{2}$ teaspoon ginger, minced
1 teaspoon vanilla extract
Dash of cinnamon (optional)

Add all the ingredients to a blender and blend until smooth.

EGG-BASED BREAKFASTS

Bacon and Egg Scramble Cakes

Servings: 5   Cheats/Serving: 2

These freeze well: Try freezing leftovers in individual plastic bags to easily reheat them later.

1 tablespoon olive or coconut oil
5 pieces grass-fed or nitrate-free bacon, chopped
3 shallots, chopped
5 omega 3–enriched eggs
1 handful parsley, chopped
Fresh berries for serving

Preheat oven to 350 degrees F.

Heat the oil in a skillet over medium heat. Once the skillet is hot, fry the bacon and shallots for 4 minutes.

Meanwhile, whip the eggs in a bowl for at least 45 seconds. Add the bacon, shallots, and parsley to the eggs and mix with a fork.

Pour the mixture into muffin tins, until they are nearly full. Bake for 20 minutes or until the eggs are set.Serve with berries.

Meg's Mexican Breakfast Skillet

Servings: 1   **Cheats/Serving: 2**

This recipe pairs wonderfully with sautéed kale, spinach, or collard greens.

1/2 tablespoon olive oil
1 cup organic hash browns
2 eggs
1/2 cup black beans
3/4 cup salsa (you can use as much as you want, really)
1/4 cup salsa verde (optional)

Have a small and a large saucepan (with a cover) on the stove. Heat the large saucepan on high until hot. Add the olive oil and hash browns. Cover for 3 minutes, flip hash browns, and cover again.

After the hash browns have been flipped, heat the small saucepan on medium. When the pan is hot, crack eggs and cook on medium. I like eggs over easy, but you can cook them any way you'd like.

When the hash browns have cooked another 3 minutes, mix so that whichever side is less done is on the pan side. Add the black beans. When the black beans have heated up, add the salsa and salsa verde. When the salsa has warmed, take off the heat and put on a plate. Top with the cooked eggs.

Nearly Cheat-Free Huevos Rancheros with Spicy Garlic Kale

Servings: 1   **Cheats/Serving: 2.5**

1 tablespoon olive oil
1 garlic clove, minced or pressed (add more if you love garlic)
4 cup kale
1 cup water
½ cup black beans (optional)
2 eggs
1 cup salsa
Adobo seasoning to taste
Red pepper flakes to taste
Salt and pepper to taste

Heat olive oil in a sauté or saucepan over medium heat. When the oil is warm but not hot, add garlic. Once you can smell the garlic, add the kale and water, and cover.

While the kale is cooking, heat the black beans and scramble the eggs in a separate bowl. When the eggs are scrambled, top them with a shake of adobo.

Heat a small pan over medium-high heat and begin to cook the eggs. When the kale is done cooking, add red pepper flakes, salt, and pepper and combine with the eggs.

Simply Divine Egg, Bacon, and Goat Cheese Omelet

Servings: 1   **Cheats/Serving: 3**

To make this even faster in the morning, use leftover stir-fry vegetables instead of the vegetables as an omelet from the night before!

1 teaspoon olive oil or butter
¼ sweet yellow onion, thinly sliced

2 garlic cloves
8 mushrooms, sliced
1 cup organic spinach
Salt and pepper to taste
2 eggs
Bacon and goat cheese confetti

Heat a skillet over medium heat. Once heated, add the oil. Add the onions and cook until they're light brown. Add the garlic and cook for about a minute. Add the mushrooms and sauté for 4 minutes, and then add the spinach and cook for another minute. Season with salt and pepper. Remove the vegetables from the pan and set aside.

In a small bowl, stir the eggs until they're smooth. Add them to the same skillet and cook until the eggs are almost cooked like a pancake. Add the vegetable mixture and the confetti on top, and then fold over the eggs to create your omelet.

South of the Border Eggs

Servings: 1   **Cheats/Serving: 2.5**

2 hard-boiled eggs, chopped
¼ avocado, chopped
Tomato and jalapeño dip or organic salsa to taste

Mix ingredients in a small bowl.

POWER BREAKFASTS

Power Workout Breakfast

Servings: 1   **Cheats/Serving: 1**

1 teaspoon olive oil
⅓ sweet yellow onion, chopped
2 cups broccoli stems, chopped
1 tablespoon crushed walnuts or 1 tablespoon hemp seeds
3 handfuls fresh spinach leaves
1 tablespoon oregano
2 cups cooked lentils
1 teaspoon salt
3 basil leaves, chopped

Heat a pan over medium-high heat and add the olive oil and onions. Sauté the onions until they're brown, and then add the broccoli stems. If the pan is a bit dry at this point, add 2 tablespoons of water. Cook for 4 minutes.

Add the walnuts or hemp seeds and stir, cooking for 2 minutes. Add the spinach leaves, oregano, lentils, and salt and heat through.

Adjust the salt or oregano if needed, and garnish with basil before serving.

Scott's Summer Breakfast Salad

Servings: varies, depending on   **Cheats/Serving:**
ingredients used   **0 + 1/protein serving**

Use as much or as little of each ingredient as you like! This salad is endlessly customizable—just have fun!

Mixed greens
Fresh spinach
1 handful arugula

Chopped strawberries

Blueberries

Raspberries

Any seasonal stone fruit, chopped (peaches, pears, nectarines)

Protein of choice

Fruit-flavored balsamic vinaigrette (These are found mostly at specialty stores that carry different olive oils and vinegars.)

Toasted almonds or Cinnamon Candied Walnuts (page 287) (optional)

Combine the ingredients in a medium-sized salad bowl. (You need to add a protein so this isn't a salad-as-meal.) Top with ½ tablespoon of dressing and mix. Garnish with the almonds or walnuts.

LUNCH RECIPES

SOUPS

Beef Stroganoff Soup

Servings: 4   **Cheats/Serving: 4.5**

1 ½ pounds grass-fed ground beef or beef tenderloin (cut into ¼-inch thick slices)

1 to 2 teaspoons sea salt, to taste

1 teaspoon ground black pepper

¼ cup onion, chopped

8 ounces white mushrooms, sliced thinly

1 cup organic beef stock

½ cup coconut milk (light)

1 cup coconut cream

1 medium zucchini, julienned

1 large carrot, julienned

2 large garlic cloves, pressed in garlic press or diced

1 tablespoon Dijon mustard

Chopped fresh parsley or dill for garnishment (optional)

Lightly season the beef with salt and pepper. On medium-high heat, brown the beef and onion until meat is browned and onions are tender. Add remaining ingredients except parsley or dill.

Bring to boil, then reduce heat to low, cover, and simmer for about 10 minutes

Uncover and simmer for about 10 to 15 minutes until zucchini and carrots are to desired tenderness

Serve hot in bowls and garnish with parsley or dill, if desired.

Big Barley Soup

Servings: 4   **Cheats/Serving: 1.5**

8 cups canned low-sodium beef broth or homemade stock
1 large onion, chopped
2 medium carrots, chopped
2 celery stalks, chopped
½ cup chopped green pepper
1 cup frozen peas
⅔ cup barley
½ teaspoon tamari
1 tablespoon fresh basil, chopped, or 1 teaspoon dried basil
Salt and pepper to taste

Add all the ingredients to a slow cooker. Cook on medium heat for 3 to 4 hours.

Chicken Piccata Soup

Servings: 8   **Cheats/Serving: 2**

1 cup organic low-sodium chicken broth
½ cup lemon juice
4 skinless, boneless chicken breasts

3 tablespoons olive oil
1 onion, minced
3 cloves garlic, minced
1 cup artichoke hearts, chopped
3 tablespoons capers (optional)
1 teaspoon freshly ground pepper
1 tablespoon parsley, minced (optional for garnishment)

In a resealable food storage bag, combine broth, lemon juice, and chicken. Marinate chicken overnight.

The next day, in a medium skillet, heat oil over medium heat and sauté onion and garlic until softened, about 2 minutes. Remove chicken from bag (reserve marinade) and place in skillet to brown each side, 5 to 10 minutes. Add artichoke hearts, capers, pepper, and reserved marinade.

Reduce heat and simmer until chicken is thoroughly cooked, about 10 minutes.

Garnish with parsley, if desired, and serve.

Chilled Summer Gazpacho

Servings: 4   **Cheats/Serving: 1**

Though you can eat this about a half hour after you make it, this chilled soup is best if you let it sit in the fridge for a day so the flavors can blend together. It's the perfect summer soup.

Feel free to experiment with different vegetables as well! All you technically need to make gazpacho is tomato juice, onion, and cilantro. Everything else is up to you!

1 red bell pepper
1 yellow bell pepper
1 orange bell pepper
1 green bell pepper
2 cucumbers, peeled
2 red onions
One 28-ounce can diced tomatoes
2 garlic cloves, diced
One to two 12-ounce bottles of V8 vegetable juice (you can use
   tomato juice as well, though V8 is a better base)
Dried or fresh jalapeños, diced (optional)
Cayenne pepper to taste
Chipotle-style hot sauce
Dash sea salt and coarsely ground black pepper to taste
Adobo seasoning to taste
½ cup fresh cilantro, chopped
¼ cup fresh parsley, chopped
1 avocado

Dice the bell peppers, cucumbers, and onions to whatever size you'd like. Put bell peppers, cucumbers, onions, diced tomatoes, and garlic in a large stockpot that fits in your fridge. Add the V8 juice until the consistency of the soup is as you like it. Mix well. Add the jalapeño peppers and seasonings. This soup's taste varies a lot based on the seasonings you use, so feel free to experiment until you get the taste you want.

Once the taste is right, add the cilantro and parsley and let the soup sit in your fridge for at least a half hour; or best of all, let it sit overnight. When ready to serve, add slices of avocado to the top. Yum!

My Mom's Chili

Servings: 8   **Cheats/Serving: 1**

This chili recipe is an easy one to double or triple if you have guests.

1 tablespoon olive or coconut oil
1 pound grass-fed ground beef or ground turkey
2 tomatoes, diced
One 15-ounce can unsalted pinto beans, kept in their liquid
One 15-ounce can unsalted kidney beans, kept in their liquid
2 tablespoons minced onion
1½ teaspoons chili powder
1 teaspoon sea salt
½ teaspoon minced garlic
½ teaspoon ground cumin
½ cup water

In a frying pan over medium heat, heat the oil. Add the meat and cook until it is browned.

Mix all the ingredients together in a slow cooker. Cook on high for 2 to 3 hours, and then turn the heat down to low until you're ready to serve.

Philly Cheesesteak Soup

Servings: 4   **Cheats/Serving: 3**

1 onion, chopped
4 ounces mushrooms (optional)
1 green bell pepper, chopped
1 pound grass-fed beef stew meat, cut into thin strips
¼ teaspoon fresh ginger, minced
¼ teaspoon red pepper flakes
6 ounces of Parmesan cheese

Sauté onion and mushroom in a skillet over medium-high heat for about 2 to 3 minutes. After onion is softened, add pepper. Then add the meat, ginger, and red pepper flakes to the skillet.

Cover and cook until the meat is to your preferred tenderness. Top with Parmesan cheese until melted. Remove from heat, then serve and enjoy!

SALADS & DRESSINGS

Asian Chicken Salad

Servings: 4   **Cheats/Serving: 2**

The bok choy in this recipe is super crunchy and makes an excellent base that can support a variety of flavors. As you develop the habit of adding bok choy to your salads, you'll find yourself eating a lot of it. And one head of bok choy has around 900 milligrams of calcium! You can also add chopped spinach to this salad for more nutrients.

1 pound boneless, skinless chicken thighs
1 head bok choy
1 bunch scallions

Dressing

1 tablespoon toasted sesame oil or ½ an avocado

Juice of 1 lemon (or more to taste)

1 tablespoon honey (this is a must for the recipe)

1 teaspoon sea salt

Black pepper to taste

1 finger's worth of ginger

Crushed red pepper flakes to taste

1 jalapeño, minced (optional)

Parsley or cilantro (optional)

Almonds or almond butter

Heat the oil in a pan over medium heat. Once hot, add the chicken and cook through. Be sure to cut one piece of chicken open to ensure it's cooked throughout (it's no longer dark pink). Once cooked, drain the fat, cool, and chop. You can use all the chicken or save half in the fridge to use later in a second batch. For a vegan option, substitute tofu or some other plant-based food for the chicken.

Chop the bok choy and green onion as finely as you can. Toss them into a large bowl with the cooled chicken.

Using a food processor or blender, blend the dressing ingredients. You can really work the flavor here, and adjust to your own tastes.

Toss the dressing into the chicken mixture. If you want a spicier salad, add more spices. If you want a nuttier flavor, add more sesame oil. Top with parsley or cilantro and almonds.

Tip: If you don't have almonds, use a single serving pack of Justin's Classic Almond Nut Butter.

Avocado and Bacon Chicken Salad

Servings: 4   **Cheats/Serving: 2 + 1 Cheat Confetti serving of bacon**

1 pound grilled chicken breast (precooked, store-bought chicken works here)
1 avocado
1 lemon
Salt and pepper to taste
Cayenne pepper to taste
Cheat Confetti Bacon for garnish (recipe on page 210)

Cut the chicken and avocado into small chunks and place in a bowl. Add the juice from the lemon and stir. Add the salt, pepper, and cayenne pepper. Top with Cheat Confetti Bacon and serve.

Chaat Masala and Lime Dressing (Cheat free!)

Servings: 2   **Cheats/Serving: 0**

This recipe is courtesy of Uma Naidoo, M.D. Uma is a wonderful friend of ours who is a culinary delight. I highly encourage you to make her dressings!

You can purchase chaat masala online, at an Indian grocer.

2 tablespoons chaat masala
¼ cup fresh-squeezed lime juice
¼ cup fresh-squeezed orange juice
1 tablespoon white wine vinegar
Salt to taste
Lime zest to taste

Whisk ingredients together and store in an airtight container.

Creamy Caesar Salad Dressing

Servings: 2   **Cheats/Serving: 0.5**

Sometimes you just want the taste of Caesar dressing, but we all know it can make a large classic Caesar salad with croutons ordered at a restaurant more than 20 Cheats! Here is our version—and for those of you who are gluten-free, we've made this for you.

2 fresh anchovies
3 garlic cloves
5 heaping tablespoons low-fat Greek yogurt
3 tablespoons tamari
Juice of 1 lemon
1 tablespoon Parmesan cheese
½ teaspoon salt
Freshly ground black pepper

Roughly chop the anchovies and garlic. Add all the ingredients to a blender or food processor and blend until smooth.

Serve with romaine lettuce and grilled chicken.

Creamy Chicken Salad

Servings: 4   **Cheats/Serving: 1.5**

1 pound grilled chicken breast
4 tablespoons low-fat Greek yogurt
2 garlic cloves, minced
2 tablespoons tamari
Juice of ½ lemon
Sea salt and pepper to taste

Cut the chicken breast into ½-inch chunks and set aside.

Add the yogurt, garlic, tamari, lemon juice, sea salt, and pepper to a blender or food processor and blend until smooth.

Pour the dressing over the chicken and mix thoroughly.

Diced Chicken, Grape, and Slivered Almond Salad

Servings: 5   Cheats/Serving: 2.5

3½ cups boneless, skinless free-range chicken breasts, diced
2 teaspoons apple cider vinegar or lemon juice
½ cup light or homemade mayonnaise
10 white seedless grapes, halved
1 cup celery, diced
⅓ cup pecans, chopped, or almonds, slivered

In a pot, bring enough water to cover the chicken to a boil. Once it's boiling, add the chicken and cook for 15 to 20 minutes, or until the chicken is no longer pink in the center. Remove the chicken from the water and let it cool.

Once it's cool enough to handle, shred the meat.

In a large mixing bowl, combine all the ingredients and mix well. Serve chilled.

Green-Tea Poppy Seed Mint Vinaigrette

Servings: 4   Cheats/Serving: 0.5

Courtesy Uma Naidoo, M.D.

½ cup chilled green tea (drained of tea leaves or tea bag)
¼ cup fresh-squeezed orange juice with pulp (for texture)
2 tablespoons extra-virgin olive oil
1 tablespoon fresh mint

1 tablespoon poppy seeds
⅛ teaspoon ground ginger powder
Salt to taste
Orange zest to taste

Shake ingredients together and store in an airtight container.

Jackie's Vail Chophouse Salad

Servings: 2   **Cheats/Serving: 2**
(chicken), 3 with optional bacon

There is no extra dressing in this recipe. The avocado and lemon, along with the salt and pepper, give this salad the perfect moist consistency.

8 ounces salmon
Juice of 1 lemon or 1 lime
Salt and pepper to taste

OR

8-ounce lean chicken cutlet
1 teaspoon olive oil
Salt and pepper to taste

¼ to ½ pound mixed greens
¼ red onion, thinly sliced into half moons
½ avocado
Juice of ½ lemon (optional)
Salt and pepper to taste (optional)
5 cashews, chopped, or 1½ bacon slices, crumbled (optional)

To Make the Salmon:

Preheat the oven to 400 degrees F.

In a baking dish, place a sheet of parchment paper large enough to wrap the salmon. Place the salmon on the parchment paper. Add lemon juice, salt, and pepper on top. Seal the parchment paper around the salmon. Bake for 22 minutes, checking the fish after 15 minutes. It's done when it is easily flaked with a fork.

To Make the Chicken:

Place a saucepan over medium heat. Add the olive oil.

Slice the chicken into pieces with a chicken shears. Place the chicken in the pan and add salt and pepper. Cook 4 minutes each side until the chicken is no longer pink when cut open.

To Assemble the Salad:

In very large mixing bowl, add the greens, onion, avocado, lemon juice, salt, and pepper, and cashews or bacon, if desired. Mix well. Add the warm salmon or chicken and mix.

Jicama, Grapefruit, and Cilantro Salad

Servings: 2   Cheats/Serving: 0

You can substitute 2 mangoes for the grapefruit in this recipe.

1 large jicama, peeled and cut into 2-inch long strips
2 small red onion, thinly sliced into rings
2 red grapefruits, peeled and segmented with membranes removed
Juice of 1 lime
2 tablespoons cilantro, chopped
Sea salt to taste
Cayenne pepper to taste

In a large bowl, gently mix all the ingredients. Chill before serving.

Julie's Taco Salad

Servings: 6   **Cheats/Serving: 3**

Julie was a college roommate of mine and she is obsessed with perfecting the Taco Salad. This is her best!

1 pound ground turkey meat
1 small package (approximately 1 ounce) of organic taco seasoning
½ cup (8 ounces) Catalina dressing
One 15-ounce can of kidney beans, drained
1 head of lettuce, chopped or torn into small pieces
1 tomato, chopped
8 ounces shredded cheddar cheese
Tortilla chips, crushed
1 8-ounce jar of salsa, or more to taste (optional)

Brown the turkey in a skillet over medium heat. Drain the meat, put it back into the skillet, and add the taco seasoning and the Catalina dressing. Stir well. Add the kidney beans and then set the mixture aside.

Prepare the salad by layering the lettuce and meat and kidney bean mixture in a bowl. Add the tomato and cheese. Mix. Now add the desired amount of crushed tortilla chips on top. Serve with salsa on the side to add as dressing, if desired.

Lemon Almond Miso Sauce

Servings: 8 **Cheats/Serving: 0.5**

This sauce is wonderful with any protein, or even as a dressing on mixed greens.

4 heaping tablespoons almond butter
2 heaping tablespoon miso (any color)
3½ cups water, for thinning
1 lemon

In a saucepan over medium heat, add the almond butter, miso, water, and lemon zest. Whisk until integrated, 5 to 10 minutes. Add the juice from the lemon and mix.

Lemon Wasabi Dressing

Servings: 1 **Cheats/Serving: 0**

This dressing is wonderful on fish.

Juice of 2 lemons
1 teaspoon wasabi
1 teaspoon tamari

Mix together all the ingredients and then serve.

Magic Lime Dressing

Servings: 1 **Cheats/Serving: 0**

Juice of 2 limes
Salt to taste
4 shakes red pepper flakes

Add ingredients to a small bowl and mix well.

The Mediterranean Espagna Salad

Servings: 1   **Cheats/Serving: 2**

The "Med" is one of our favorite go-to restaurants in Boulder and this happens to be one of their best salads!

Field greens
¼ cucumber, chopped
6 grape tomatoes (halved)
4 strawberries, sliced
1 tablespoon toasted pine nuts
1 tablespoon red onion, minced
Magic Lime Dressing
Protein of choice
1 ounce goat cheese

Toss the greens, cucumber, tomatoes, strawberries, pine nuts, and red onion in a bowl. Add the dressing and toss well to coat. Top the salad with your favorite protein and goat cheese.

Mexican City Chicken Salad

Servings: 4   **Cheats/Serving: 1.5**

1 pound grilled chicken breast
½ pound pico de gallo (recipe below, or use store-bought)
1 cup black beans (optional)

Pico de Gallo

1 tomato
¼ red onion
¼ jalapeño
¼ avocado
2 tablespoons cilantro
Juice of ½ lime

Cut the chicken breast into small chunks and place in a medium-sized bowl. If you're using store-bought pico de gallo, add that to the bowl, and then add the black beans. Mix well.

If you're making your own pico de gallo, finely dice the tomato, onion, and jalapeño. Mix them together in a small bowl. Dice the avocado and add it and the cilantro to the bowl. Squeeze the lime juice over the tomato mixture and then mix well.

Moong Dal Salad

Servings: 2   **Cheats/Serving: 0**

Substitute other sprouted beans for moong beans if you wish. Split moong beans are available in health food stores or in Indian grocery stores.

1 cup split yellow moong beans
1 tomato, chopped
1 cucumber, peeled and chopped
3 to 4 red radishes, chopped
½ red onion or 3 to 4 scallions, chopped
2 tablespoons fresh ginger, minced
½ jalapeño, minced
3 tablespoons lemon juice
½ cup cilantro, chopped
Sea salt to taste

Rinse the beans in several changes of water and soak for at least an hour in 3 cups of water.

Drain the beans and place in a serving dish. Add the remaining ingredients and mix thoroughly.

Night Eater's Best Friend Salad

Servings: 3   **Cheats/Serving: 1**

This salad is designed for eating between 4 and 6 P.M. It contains a ton of micronutrients. Ideally, you'll eat the bulk of this yourself, but share if you must. In our experience, it is impossible to make too much salad. If you have someone in your home who is not a salad eater, this is a great way to convert them to the power of a massive salad.

Because this salad is delicious, it helps you realize that eating high volumes of greens can be done easily. As our friend Dr. Joel Fuhrman says, the salad is the main course. This one is awesome if you like a crunchy, flavorful eating experience.

3 hearts of romaine lettuce
2 handfuls salad mix: spring mix, herb mix, or baby spinach
½ avocado
Juice of 1 lemon
1 teaspoon Grey Poupon Dijon Mustard
2 garlic cloves, crushed and diced
1 tablespoon olive oil
Salt and pepper to taste
Cheat Confetti of your choice

Chop the 3 romaine hearts into ½-inch strips and place in a large bowl. Add your salad mix of choice. Dice the avocado and add it to the bowl. In a small bowl, whisk together the remaining ingredients (except for the Cheat Confetti) until emulsified.

Mix the dressing from the small bowl into your salad greens, and then top with your Cheat Confetti.

Pear and Roquefort Salad

Servings: 4   **Cheats/Serving: 1**

1 red pear
1 green pear
½ red onion, sliced
1 tablespoon Roquefort cheese
1 handful walnuts
Freshly chopped parsley to taste

Dressing
Juice of 1 lemon
1 drop good mustard
1 drop good honey (organic when possible)
½ tablespoon olive oil

Wash the fruit, and then slice the pears and place them on a plate, alternating colors. Add onion slices. Top with cheese, walnuts, and parsley.

In a small bowl, combine the dressing ingredients and whisk until the dressing thickens. Pour over the pears.

Savory Rosemary Chicken Salad

Servings: 4   **Cheats/Serving: 2**

If you're buying the chicken fresh from the counter or butcher, ask them to cut it into squares or strips for you. Just mention you're making a stir-fry or salad and they'll be happy to do it. This saves a ton of time for you when you're preparing this dish.

1½ pounds mixed greens
1 tablespoon freeze-dried dill or 1 fresh dill sprig
3 tablespoons fresh cilantro (optional)
3 tablespoons Italian parsley

½ tablespoon olive or coconut oil
1 pound lean, organic chicken cutlets
3 fresh rosemary sprigs or 2 tablespoons fresh rosemary
3 tablespoons sliced red onion
½ avocado
Sea salt and pepper to taste
Juice of ½ lemon or 2 tablespoons apple cider vinegar

In a large salad bowl, mix the greens, dill, cilantro, and parsley.

In a saucepan over medium heat, add the olive or coconut oil and then the chicken. Add the rosemary, spreading it evenly over the chicken. Cook 8 to 10 minutes, flipping 3 to 4 times during the cooking with tongs. Be sure to cut a piece of chicken open to make sure it's cooked throughout (no longer dark pink). Set the chicken aside.

Add the onions, avocado, chicken, salt, and pepper to the mixed greens. Add the lemon juice and mix well.

Simple French Dijon Dressing

Servings: 2   **Cheats/Serving: 1**

1 tablespoon of Dijon (no honey, no spice, straight Dijon)
Juice of 2 lemons
2 garlic cloves, chopped
2 tablespoons olive oil
Pinch of salt

Blend all of the ingredients together.

Tequila-Pineapple Dressing

Servings: 2   **Cheats/Serving: 0.5**

Courtesy Uma Naidoo, M.D.

For a nonalcoholic version of this dressing, substitute apple cider vinegar for the tequila. This will also lower the calorie count.

1 ounce tequila
¼ cup lime juice
½ cup lemon sparkling water
½ cup fresh pineapple purée
Salt to taste

Combine ingredients in an airtight container.

Tex-Mex Salad with Potato Chips

Servings: 1   **Cheats/Serving: 2.5**

This is my favorite salad, even after years of eating it! The best part is the Tex-Mex Tabbouleh. In addition to using it for this salad, I use it for a ton of other recipes since it's delicious and completely cheat-free.

If you don't have the ingredients for the Tex-Mex Tabbouleh, just combine salsa or pico de gallo with 2 cups of quinoa.

4 huge handfuls mixed greens, chopped
¼ head cabbage, chopped
½ cup fresh or canned chickpeas (optional)
1 cup of Tex-Mex Tabbouleh (recipe to follow)
½ avocado
Juice of 2 limes
Salt to taste

Red pepper flakes to taste
1 gigantic handful plain sea salt potato chips (optional)

Place the mixed greens and cabbage in a bowl. Add the chickpeas, Tex-Mex Tabbouleh, avocado, juice of 2 limes, salt, and red pepper flakes. Crumble the potato chips on top, if desired, and toss well.

Tex-Mex Tabbouleh

Servings: 4   Cheats/Serving: 0

2 cups cooked quinoa
1 tomato, chopped
1 cucumber, halved and seeds removed, and then chopped
3 tablespoons red onions or scallions, chopped
½ jalapeño, chopped (optional)
Juice of ½ lime
2 tablespoons cilantro
Salt to taste

Mix together the quinoa, tomato, cucumber, red onions, and jalapeño. Add the lime juice and cilantro and mix well. Add salt.

Watermelon-Mint-Caper Dressing (Cheat free!)

Courtesy Uma Naidoo, M.D.

Servings: 4   Cheats/Serving: 0

½ cup watermelon juice (blend seedless watermelon to make fresh juice)
½ cup sparkling water
2 tablespoons capers, puréed
1 tablespoon mint, chopped
Kosher salt to taste
Pinch of black salt

Combine ingredients in an airtight container.

CHEAT CONFETTI FOR LUNCH

Cheat Confetti Bacon

Servings: 4   **Cheats/Serving: 1**

Try to find organic and uncured bacon for this recipe.

4 bacon strips, sliced in half

Place a large saucepan over medium heat. Take the 8 half-strips of bacon and place in the saucepan. Every few minutes, flip until the strips are a crispy golden brown. Be sure not to burn the bacon! You have to be in the kitchen when you're cooking these.

Once crisp, remove from the pan and place on doubled paper towels. Blot any extra grease. Crumble each strip into small pieces and place into a small airtight container. Serve atop your favorite salad or dish as Cheat Confetti.

Cheat Confetti Parmesan Crisps

Servings: 4   **Cheats/Serving: 0.5**

Use these as confetti atop salads, chicken, or your favorite casserole. Double this recipe if you'd like to keep extra for your magic fridge.

10 tablespoons shredded Parmesan cheese

Place a small saucepan over medium heat. When it's hot, spread shredded Parmesan as evenly as possible in the pan. Do not stir or flip. When the Parmesan is light brown and an almost solid sheet, remove it with a spatula. Let it cool, and then break it up into pieces.

Power Green Confetti

Servings: 4   **Cheats/Serving: 0**

This Cheat-free confetti adds greens to any dish without compromising the taste. Serve with salad, soup or any favorite dish for color or as herbs.

½ pound greens (kale, spinach, whatever you like)
Favorite herbs (optional)

Put your washed greens and any herbs you'd like into a food processor. Process until they're finely chopped.

PROTEIN BASED AND MORE

The Basalt

Servings: 4   **Cheats/Serving: 2.5**

The perfect answer to your bacon, lettuce, and tomato sandwich, Cheatified.

---

3 cooked bacon strips
1 pound cooked salmon
1 tomato, sliced
Arugula or mixed greens
Very large romaine hearts
Pico de gallo or PEERtrainer Spicy Ranch Dressing (page 282)

Layer the bacon, salmon, tomato, and arugula on large romaine hearts or large cabbage leaves. Add pico de gallo or the ranch dressing.

Chipotle Shrimp Fajitas with Avocado and Salsa

Servings: 4   **Cheats/Serving: 1.5 with the optionals**

1 tablespoon olive oil
1 pound large shrimp, deveined and peeled
Chipotle seasoning to taste
Red pepper flakes to taste
2 red onions, sliced
1 green pepper, sliced
1 red pepper, sliced
½ cups mushrooms, sliced (optional)
½ jalapeño, sliced (optional)
Adobo seasoning to taste
Boston lettuce
Salsa (optional)
Avocado, diced (optional)
Black beans (optional)

Heat a skillet over medium heat. Add the olive oil. Coat the shrimp in chipotle seasoning and place in the hot pan. After 1 to 2 minutes, add the red pepper flakes, onions, peppers, mushrooms, and jalapeños.

When the shrimp is no longer translucent and the vegetables have softened, add the adobo seasoning and heat through.

Create wraps with the Boston lettuce leaves, shrimp mixture, and salsa, avocado, or black beans.

Classic Italian Grilled Cheese

Servings: 1   **Cheats/Serving: 4**

1 teaspoon olive oil
1½ slices sharp cheddar cheese
1 teaspoon dried Italian seasoning or dried oregano
2 slices of your favorite bread

Place a frying pan over medium heat. Add the olive oil to the pan. Prepare the sandwich by placing the cheese and herbs on one slice of bread, then placing the other slice of bread on top.

Cook the sandwich in the frying pan until the bread is toasted and the cheese is melted, flipping the sandwich over at least once to toast both slices of bread.

Easy Foil Rosemary Chicken

Servings: 2   **Cheats/Serving: 1**

1 chicken breast
4 fresh rosemary sprigs
Salt and pepper to taste

Preheat oven to 350 degrees F.

Take two sprigs of rosemary and pull the leaves off the stem. Chop in quarters if possible (halves are okay, too).

Place a piece of foil that will cover the chicken in a baking dish; place half of the rosemary underneath the chicken breast and then sprinkle the top with salt and pepper. Add the remaining half of the rosemary to the top of the chicken and seal the foil.

Bake for 30 minutes.

Easy Italian Herb Baked Turkey

Servings: 4   **Cheats/Serving: 1**

1 pound organic, boneless turkey breast
1 teaspoon oil
1 lemon or 1 lime
1 handful fresh herbs (basil and oregano)
1 teaspoon salt

Preheat oven to 350 degrees F.

Set aside a piece of tinfoil large enough to completely wrap the turkey breast.

Rub the turkey breast with oil. Place it on one side of the tinfoil. Slice the lemon or lime and lay the slices on top of the turkey breast. Place the fresh herbs on top of the lemon or lime.

Fold the tinfoil and roll the edges like a calzone.

Bake on a cookie sheet or in a baking dish for 25 to 35 minutes.

Eggplant, Tomato, and Mozzarella Italian Casserole

Servings: 4   **Cheats/Serving: 1 Cheat per serving**

1 eggplant
1 large ripe tomato
4 ounces fresh mozzarella
One 24-ounce jar tomato sauce (organic or simple marinara or basil)
Fresh basil to taste

Preheat oven to 350 degrees F.

Peel the eggplant and then slice it into thin rounds. Slice the tomato and mozzarella into rounds.

In a baking dish, cover the bottom with the tomato sauce.

Layer one slice of eggplant, one slice of tomato, and one slice of mozzarella and place it in the dish, being careful to keep each tower separate. When you've finished your towers, top them with the fresh basil and a little more sauce.

Bake for 35 minutes.

Fresh Spring Green Beans with Slivered Almonds

Servings: 2 **Cheats/Serving: 1**

1 pound fresh green beans, trimmed
1/2 teaspoon salt, divided
1 teaspoon coconut oil
2 green onions, chopped
1/4 cup slivered almonds or pecans

Bring 1½ inches of water to a boil in a medium pot fitted with a steamer basket.

Sprinkle green beans with ¼ teaspoon salt and place in the steamer basket. Cover and steam for 10 minutes, or until the green beans are tender-crisp.

Immediately plunge the green beans into an ice-water bath to stop the cooking, and then drain them.

Meanwhile, heat a nonstick skillet over medium-high heat. Add the oil once the pan is hot. Add the green onions and sauté 2 to 3 minutes, or until they're soft. Add the green beans, nuts, and remaining salt, stirring until thoroughly heated.

Hot and Spicy Black Beans and Rice

Servings: 4 **Cheats/Serving: 0**

1 tablespoon olive oil
3/4 cup onion, chopped
1/2 green pepper, chopped
1 cup tomatoes, diced
One 15-ounce can black beans (drained but reserve the liquid)
1/2 teaspoon thyme
1 teaspoon garlic, minced
3 tablespoons apple cider vinegar
1/2 teaspoon hot sauce
1 cup of white or black rice

In a skillet over medium heat, heat the olive oil. Once the oil is hot, cook the onion and green pepper until they are tender. Stir in the tomatoes, drained beans, thyme, and garlic. Cook for 3 minutes.

Add the vinegar, hot sauce, and reserved bean liquid. Cook for 5 more minutes. Serve over rice. Enjoy!

Mediterranean Gourmet Power Bowl

Servings: 4   **Cheats/Serving: 0.5 (1 with "Optionals")**

Mediterranean cuisine is one of my favorites. It feels so fresh and clean and tastes like spring. I created this after spotting a great advertisement by Udi's for their sun-dried tomato and artichoke pizza.

In this recipe, if you'd like to be extra fancy, you can roast 8 garlic cloves at 400 degrees F for 25 minutes instead of using the 3 cloves of chopped garlic.

1½ cups uncooked quinoa (approximately 4 cups cooked)
One 14-ounce can or jar artichoke hearts
15 sun-dried tomatoes, quartered
Spinach, kale, or bok choy finely chopped in a food processor (enough to help reach a daily goal of ½ pound of greens) (optional)
2 tablespoons extra-virgin olive oil
3 garlic cloves, chopped
½ cup fresh basil
3 shakes crushed red pepper (or more to taste)
Salt to taste
1 ounce goat cheese, crumbled (optional)

Prepare quinoa according to the package directions. It's usually 1 cup of quinoa to 2 cups of water. I highly recommend preparing in the rice cooker. If you don't have a rice cooker, just bring the water to a boil, add the quinoa, reduce the heat, cover, and simmer for 15 to 17 minutes until it is fluffy.

While quinoa is cooking, place artichoke hearts, sun-dried tomatoes, spinach or other greens, olive oil, garlic, basil, and red pepper flakes in mixing bowl. When quinoa is ready, add it to bowl, and then add a pinch of salt and goat cheese, if desired.

Microwave No-Time Salmon with Broccoli

Servings: 1   **Cheats/Serving: 1.5**

1 frozen dinner with salmon that contains 4 ounces of salmon
One 16-ounce package frozen broccoli
Lemon juice to taste

Open the frozen dinner and discard any Cheat you don't want (rice, pasta, etc.).

Open the broccoli and place it on top of your frozen dinner. Heat the salmon and broccoli until fully cooked, and then sprinkle with lemon juice.

Mojo Cuban Rub Salmon

Servings: 4   **Cheats/Serving: 1.5**

As crazy as this sounds, if you're intimidated by the oven or saucepan, you can cook this in the microwave. I'll give you both the oven and microwave versions.

Please do not get Atlantic farmed salmon for this recipe. Yes, it probably tastes better because it's fattier, but with these spices, you're really going to start liking wild salmon. I prefer Coho.

1 pound organic wild salmon
2 tablespoons Whole Foods Mojo Cuban Rub spice
Salt and pepper to taste

Oven directions:

Preheat oven to 400 degrees F. Place salmon on parchment paper or foil, add the Mojo Cuban Rub spice, salt, and pepper. Wrap the fish into a package and place on a cookie sheet or pan. Bake for 20 minutes. (Depending on thickness, check after 15 minutes. It should easily come apart with a butter knife.)

Microwave directions:

Place salmon in microwave-friendly dish (do not use plastic or metal). Add the Mojo Cuban Rub, salt, and pepper. Cover with a lid or dish. Microwave for 5 minutes.

Be careful, you might have a mess in your microwave if you don't cover it correctly, but sometimes it's worth not having to use the oven.

PEERtrainer Bacon Avocado Burgers

Servings: 4   Cheats/Serving: 3

Serve these burgers with a large salad with Dijon or balsamic vinaigrette (remember, each portion is the large salad bowl that you usually serve for the family) or a baked sweet potato.

1 pound grass-fed beef, divided into 4 patties
1 teaspoon olive oil
1 sweet onion, thinly sliced
1 pound button mushrooms
1 garlic clove, minced
Sea salt and pepper to taste
4 servings bacon confetti (recipe page 210)
1 avocado, sliced

Heat a large skillet over medium heat. Place the burger patties in the skillet and cover. Monitor and flip the burgers every 5 minutes or so to desired doneness.

While the burgers are cooking, in large saucepan over medium heat, add the olive oil. Add the onions, mixing slowly. Do not leave the onions! Cook for around 8 minutes, until the onions are medium amber in color. Add the mushrooms and cook until they're lightly browned. Add the garlic, salt and pepper, and bacon confetti. (Two half strips is one Cheat.)

Salmon and Cucumber Wraps

Servings: 6   **Cheats/Serving: 1**

Juice of 1 lemon
1 pound smoked salmon
1 large cucumber, peeled
¼ pound arugula, spinach or mixed greens
Capers (optional)

Squeeze lemon juice over the salmon. Using a vegetable peeler, thinly slice oblong pieces of cucumber. Next, place a slice of salmon and a bit of arugula inside the cucumber and add a few capers on top. Now wrap the cucumber around the salmon, greens, and capers and place a toothpick through the bundle to hold it together. Repeat until you've used all your ingredients.

Tangy Tenderloin

Servings: 4 (with a 1-pound tenderloin)   **Cheats/Serving: 3**

½ cup fresh-squeezed lime juice
½ teaspoon coarse sea salt
¼ onion, minced
3 garlic cloves, minced
⅓ cup pure raw unfiltered honey
⅛ teaspoon pepper
1 pound pork tenderloin
2 tablespoons olive or coconut oil

Mix all the ingredients except the pork and oil in a resealable food storage bag. Add the pork to the bag and coat well. Place in the refrigerator overnight, turning occasionally.

Preheat oven to 425 degrees F.

Remove the pork from the bag, discarding the remaining marinade.

Head a skillet over medium-high heat. Add the oil. Once the oil is hot, add the pork and sear each side until it's brown. Roast the pork in the oven 15 to 20 minutes. Check to make sure it's fully cooked and serve.

Tequila Lime Chicken

Servings: 4   **Cheats/Serving: 1.5**

½ tablespoon olive or coconut oil
1 pound organic chicken breast, precut
2 tablespoons Whole Foods Tequila Lime Blend spice
Salt and pepper to taste
½ lime (optional)

Heat a saucepan over medium heat. Add oil and then add chicken. Add spice, salt, and pepper, making sure to spread it evenly. Cook 8 to 10 minutes, flipping 3 to 4 times during cooking with tongs. Be sure to cut one piece of chicken open to ensure it's cooked throughout (it's no longer dark pink). Squeeze ½ lime over the chicken if desired.

Tunatastic with Lemon and Garlic

Servings: 4   **Cheats/Serving: 2**

This is a great topping for mixed greens.

1 pound canned tuna
Juice of 1 large lemon

1 tablespoon olive oil
1 teaspoon balsamic vinegar
1 garlic clove, minced
Sea salt and pepper to taste

Add all the ingredients to a large bowl and mix well.

Wild-Caught Tilapia with Baby Spinach, Tomatoes, and Herbs

Servings: 4   **Cheats/Serving: 1**

Cheat per 3-ounce tilapia filet

8 to 12 ounces baby spinach
Salt and pepper to taste
¼ teaspoon onion powder
¼ cup homemade or low-sodium chicken broth
Four 3-ounce wild-caught tilapia fillets
4 scallions, chopped
1 small tomato, chopped
2 tomatoes, sliced

Preheat oven to 350 degrees F.

Spray a baking dish with cooking spray or coat it with oil.

Add the spinach to the baking dish, and then sprinkle it with salt, pepper, and onion powder. Add the chicken broth.

Sprinkle the fish with salt and pepper, and then place the fish on top of the spinach. Sprinkle with the scallions and chopped tomato.

Cover the baking dish with foil and bake 20 to 25 minutes, or until the fish flakes easily with a fork.

Serve with the sliced tomatoes.

Wild-Caught Fish with Olive Oil and Paprika Vegetables

Servings: 4   **Cheats/Serving: 1 Cheat per 3-ounce white fish filet**

Four 3-ounce wild-caught whitefish fillets
2 white onions, sliced
2 cups fresh or frozen broccoli, cauliflower, and carrot mix
Olive oil
1/8 teaspoon paprika
Salt and pepper to taste

Preheat oven to 350 degrees F.

Cut 4 pieces of tinfoil, each large enough to wrap one fish fillet. Place the fish on top of the foil. Add the onion and vegetable mixture on top of the fish. Drizzle each packet with olive oil and sprinkle with paprika, salt, and pepper.

Fold the foil into packets and place them on a baking sheet. Bake for 10 to 15 minutes.

Za'atar Grilled Chicken Strips

Servings: 4   **Cheats/Serving: 1.5**

1/2 tablespoon olive or coconut oil
1 pound organic chicken breast, precut
2 tablespoons Whole Foods Za'atar spice
1/2 teaspoon cayenne pepper
Salt and pepper to taste

Heat a saucepan over medium heat. Add oil and then add chicken. Add Za'atar spice, cayenne pepper, and salt and pepper, making sure to spread it evenly. Cook 8 to 10 minutes, flipping 3 to 4 times during cooking with tongs. Be sure to cut one piece of chicken open to ensure it's cooked throughout (it's no longer dark pink). These strips make a great addition to a salad.

DINNER RECIPES

SOUPS

Best Cream of Spinach Soup

Servings: 8   **Cheats/Serving: 1**

One 13.5-ounce can unsweetened coconut milk
1½ pounds frozen or fresh spinach
4 garlic cloves, chopped
Salt and pepper to taste
Cayenne pepper or red pepper flakes to taste
¼ cup chardonnay (optional)
½ apple, chopped (optional)

In a pot over medium-high heat, add all the ingredients and bring it to a boil.

Once the soup comes to a boil, remove it from the heat. With an immersion blender, blend the soup until it's smooth.

Black Bean and Salsa Shortcut Soup

Servings: 6   **Cheats/Serving: 0,**
                                                     1 if you do "Optionals"

This can be a very easy recipe to make. If you look at any (good) black bean soup recipe, there is usually a long list of vegetables and spices. By using salsa and a curry or spice mix like Muchi Curry Powder (or any other high-quality curry powder), you can make this recipe very quickly.

Like any recipe we outline, there are many different directions you can take. We have outlined the base ingredients that you need to successfully make the recipe. We also include a list of possible ingredients that you can use to customize the soup to match your tastes.

If you don't want bacon, you can easily remove the bacon. If you have a family that includes men who wonder "where the real food is," you can up the bacon and maybe even add chunks of meat to make it more of a stew. This recipe includes plenty of nutrient-dense foods, serving the dual purpose of providing big doses of "good stuff" while also seeming like "real food."

Delivery is everything when introducing new healthy recipes and dinners in the home. When asked what's for dinner, if you answer black beans, salsa, and quinoa, invariably the answer becomes "Where's the beef?" or "That's bird food. How am I supposed to feel full?"

Always lead with the traditional ingredient. In this black bean soup, say, "We're having bacon [or chicken or steak, whatever you've added]." As long as everyone feels they are having a traditional protein, they don't anticipate dinners as this new healthy kick you're on, counting down the days until you revert back to beef Bolognese. When you answer, "A new beef dish!" or "A special chicken hungry-man chili," they start to look forward to what's next.

2 cups cooked black beans

2 to 3 cups water

½ serrano or jalapeño chili pepper (onions are a nice replacement if you like flavor but not too much spice)

One 16-ounce container of salsa

Muchi Curry or any favorite curry powder to taste

Optional Ingredients

¼ to ½ cup uncooked quinoa (or ½ to 1 cup cooked if you already have it in your fridge)

2 slices bacon

Chicken, beef, or other protein, cut into large chunks

2 cups cooked and blended kale (Thanks to Jennifer Stewart for the suggestion on our Facebook page, who said, "You can't even tell the kale is in there.")

Any extra vegetables you want or have on hand, cut into large chunks
2 tablespoons olive, coconut, or flaxseed oil (especially if you are an
  athlete)

Add the beans and water to a stockpot on the stovetop. Chop the
peppers (or onions) and add them to the water and the beans. Bring
the mixture to a boil, and then add the salsa and curry powder. From
here, this is really a "choose your own adventure" recipe. Add quinoa
if you want to make a thicker soup or stew. Add some well-cooked
bacon for some added flavor and texture. Add chicken or beef if that is
a direction you want to head. Toss in vegetables or a couple of tablespoons of oil. It's up to you.

Important Note: We strongly encourage you to follow Jennifer's
suggestion and add blended kale. Kale and other greens are very high
in nutrients that most of us don't get enough of. For example, kale
contains the highest concentration of vitamin K of any food. Vitamin K
is critical for bone health and healthy aging, yet experts say that poor
intake of vitamin K is common.

We are focusing on this because (1) the average American eats
very few greens and (2) greens contain the highest concentration of
vitamin K. Other excellent sources of vitamin K include spinach,
Swiss chard, and collard greens.

Butternut Squash Soup

Servings: 8   **Cheats/Serving: 1**
                                    (if using optional coconut milk);
                                    0 (if not)

The quality of the squash will make this soup just okay or great. Combine this soup with your favorite protein.

1 onion
1 teaspoon olive oil
1 medium to large butternut squash
1 apple
7 to 8 cups cold water
One 13.5-ounce can unsweetened coconut milk (optional)
2 to 3 teaspoons sea salt
Black pepper to taste (optional)
Fresh herbs (optional)
Lemon juice (optional)

Peel and cut the onion into quarters.

Heat a stockpot over medium heat and add the oil. When it's hot, add the onion. While the onion browns, peel the squash and cut it into large pieces. Add the squash to the stockpot, letting it brown with the onion.

Peel and quarter the apple, and then add it to the pan.

Add the water, coconut milk, and salt to the stockpot. Cook until everything is soft, about 30 minutes.

Blend with an immersion blender until smooth. Garnish with pepper, herbs, and a squeeze of lemon juice, if desired.

Carrot Ginger Soup

Servings: 10   **Cheats/Serving: 1**

12 carrots, roughly chopped
4 cups chicken broth
1 bay leaf (optional)
One 13.5-ounce can unsweetened coconut milk
1 large yellow onion, chopped
1 tablespoon olive oil
2-inch chunk fresh ginger, chopped
7 garlic cloves, minced
Juice of 2 limes
Crushed red pepper flakes to taste
1 handful cilantro, chopped
Salt to taste

Place the carrots, broth, bay leaf, and coconut milk in a large stockpot over high heat. Once boiling, turn down to a simmer.

In a large skillet over medium heat, sauté the onion in the olive oil until translucent and slightly soft and golden. Add the ginger and garlic and cook for just another minute or so. Add the onions, ginger, and garlic to the stockpot.

After the mixture has come back to a boil, turn it down and simmer for 18 minutes. Remove the bay leaf, and using an immersion blender, purée until smooth.

In a small saucepan, add the lime juice, red pepper flakes, and cilantro, and sauté over high heat for a few minutes. Pour this mixture into the puréed soup and again use the immersion blender to get the soup really smooth.

Add salt to taste.

Chicken Pho Energy Soup

Servings: 8   **Cheats/Serving: 1**

This is a variation of the PEERtrainer Energy Soup that we have been making for years. This variation takes less time, and has a very different taste and color. I find it very easy to make in the morning. It usually lasts two days.

I add a bit of salad or spinach or whatever fresh greens I have in the fridge, but this is optional if you don't have them. Additionally, the greens really alter the flavor of the soup. For a more greens-based soup, definitely check out the PEERtrainer Energy Soup recipe.

1/2 large head organic cauliflower
10 shiitake mushrooms (or 1 box of regular button mushrooms, washed)
3 large heads organic broccoli (only 1/2 the stems)
One 13.5-ounce can unsweetened coconut milk
32 ounces Pacific Organic Soup Starters Chicken Pho Soup Base
5 shakes of red pepper flakes (start with 2 shakes and increase from there to desired heat level)
3 dashes sea salt
Freshly ground pepper to taste

Place the cauliflower, mushrooms, and broccoli in a large pot. Add the coconut milk and chicken pho soup base to the pot. Bring to a boil over high heat.

Once the soup is boiling, turn down the heat and simmer for 20 minutes.

Add red pepper flakes, salt, and ground pepper.

Using an immersion blender, purée the soup. Taste for seasoning, and add red pepper flakes, salt, or ground pepper as needed.

Cream of Broccoli Weight-Loss CheatCut Soup

Servings: 8   **Cheats/Serving: 1**

This soup travels wonderfully in a Thermos. Try it with the Italian Herb Goddess Chicken on page 255.

---

3 large heads broccoli (including stems)
5 garlic cloves
1 box (32 ounces) organic chicken, mushroom, or vegetable broth
One 13.5-ounce can unsweetened coconut milk
½ pound fresh spinach leaves
½ jalapeño, chopped (optional)
Sea salt and pepper to taste (optional)

Cut the broccoli into quarters and mince the garlic.

Place the broth, coconut milk, broccoli, garlic, spinach, jalapeño, salt, and pepper in a large stockpot over high heat.

When the mixture begins to boil, turn down the heat and simmer for 20 minutes.

With an immersion blender, blend the soup until it's smooth. Taste, and add more salt and pepper if needed.

Di's Hot Sausage Spice Soup

Servings: 6   **Cheats/Serving: 1**

Di is the fantastic mother of a dear friend. Her gourmet soups are often the highlight of the dinner party.

1 tablespoon olive oil
3 tablespoons basil
2 tablespoons garlic, minced
3 tablespoons fresh oregano
1 tablespoon red pepper flakes
3 scallions, chopped
1 carrot, chopped
1/2 head savoy cabbage (or more if you'd like)
2 large hot sausage links
3 1/2 cups chicken or beef stock
1 cup sliced green pepper
1 cup sliced mushrooms
1 cup peeled tomatoes, diced
1/2 cup tomato purée

Add the olive oil to a pot over medium heat. Add the basil, garlic, oregano, red pepper flakes, and scallions, and stir. Add the carrot, cabbage, and all the other ingredients. Bring to a boil, then turn down the heat and let simmer for 20 minutes.

Serve with homemade garlic and cheese croutons.

Di's Lentil Soup

Servings: 8   **Cheats/Serving: 0**

1 teaspoon olive oil
1 carrot, chopped
1 celery stalk, chopped
1 small onion, chopped
1 to 3 garlic cloves, minced

3 tomatoes, chopped (you can also use 1 small can)
2 envelopes Sazón by Goya
1 cup lentils, rinsed (green or red; I like green)
32 ounces chicken or vegetable broth, or water
2 16-ounce bags fresh or frozen spinach
Salt and pepper to taste
Red pepper flakes (optional)
Grated cheese for topping (optional)

In a stockpot, heat the olive oil over medium heat. Add the carrot, celery, onion, garlic, tomatoes, and Sazón, and then sauté for 1 minute.

Add the lentils and broth and bring to a boil. Turn the heat down to low.

Cover and cook for 30 minutes. Add the spinach and cook uncovered for 20 minutes. Add salt, pepper, and red pepper flakes. Cook 10 more minutes. Serve topped with cheese.

The Famous Puréed PEERtrainer Energy Soup

Servings: 10   **Cheats/Serving: 1**

People call and write me almost every day to tell me that they lose weight when they add this soup to their diet. If you are trying to lose weight, eat this soup before you eat other foods.

Note that unless you use an immersion blender, this recipe will be a big pain and you won't be as likely to do it. Find links on the PEERtrainer Web site for our suggested immersion blenders.

A few suggested pairings for this soup: black beans (toss them right into the soup), extra firm tofu (sauté it for 5 minutes with a bit of olive oil, sesame seeds, and red pepper flakes) or 4 ounces of baked salmon or other protein.

*4 cups chicken or vegetable broth, organic and gluten- and
preservative-free if possible*
One 13.5-ounce can unsweetened coconut milk
3 stalks broccoli (cut off the stalk ends)
*One 16-ounce bag frozen or fresh spinach (fresh gives it a beautiful
spring green color)*
One 8-ounce package of mushrooms (shiitake or a mixed box)
6 carrots
2 fresh bay leaves
1 medium yellow onion, chopped
1 tablespoon olive oil
4-inch chunk of fresh ginger, roughly chopped
6 medium garlic cloves
Juice of 2 to 3 fresh limes to taste
Crushed red pepper flakes to taste
1 handful fresh cilantro, chopped
Salt to taste

In a large stockpot over high heat, add the chicken broth and coconut milk, and then add the broccoli, spinach, mushrooms, carrots,
and bay leaves. Bring to a boil, then turn down the heat and simmer
for 18 to 20 minutes.

In a separate saucepan or large skillet over medium heat, sauté
the onions in olive oil until they are slightly soft and browned. Be
careful not to burn them.

In a food processor, grind the ginger and garlic, and then stir
them into the onions and cook for a minute. Add the onion mixture
to the broth in the stockpot.

In same pan in which you sautéed the onions, place lime juice,
crushed red pepper flakes, and the cilantro. Sauté the mixture over
high heat for 1 to 2 minutes. Add this mixture to the large stockpot.

Using an immersion blender, purée the soup until smooth. It should be a bit thick, which will help keep you satiated. Taste and add salt as needed. You can also add a bit more lime, red pepper flakes, or cilantro as needed.

Herbed Beef and Bacon Soup

Servings: 6   **Cheats/Serving: 2.5**

1 pound grass-fed ground beef

½ pound turkey bacon, grass-fed bacon, or nitrate-free bacon, cooked and crumbled

One 14.5-ounce can diced tomatoes

1 onion, chopped

1 cup celery, chopped

One 10.5-ounce can beef broth

2 cups mixed vegetables, chopped (carrots, root vegetables, greens, spinach, chard, cabbage, kale)

⅛ tablespoon dried rosemary

⅛ tablespoon dried thyme

¼ teaspoon dried basil

Salt and pepper to taste

Add all the ingredients to a slow cooker. Cook on low heat for 5 hours, or until the ground beef is thoroughly cooked.

Homemade Chicken Broth

Servings: 8 to 12   **Cheats/Serving: 0.5 per cup**

This broth is wonderful for freezing so it's available whenever a recipe calls for chicken broth.

1 whole chicken
1 onion, chopped
4 celery stalks, chopped into 4-inch pieces
4 carrots, chopped into 4-inch pieces
½ garlic bulb, cloves peeled

Place the chicken in a slow cooker and cover with cold water. Add the remaining ingredients.

Cook on low heat for 8 hours, or until the meat is tender. Separate the meat from the bones, leaving everything in the slow cooker.

Place a colander in a large bowl, and then pour the stock from the slow cooker into the colander to separate the liquid from the solids.

Insane Man Hunger Chili

Servings: 3   **Cheats/Serving: 1**

When you travel or are on the go, make a mix of this and put in containers. You can even put servings of this in a large food storage bag to keep in your jacket when you ski or are outdoors!

Salsa is the secret ingredient for this chili because it contains everything you need to make the recipe super tasty, but all you have to do is open the container into the pot! We find that the hottest salsa provides the most flavor, and dissipates once among the other ingredients.

A note on the meat: You can add more meat if you'd like, but we strongly advise spending a little more for higher quality meat. A little goes a long way, and you're getting plenty of protein from other sources. Bison and grass-fed beef don't have antibiotics or added hormones, and bison is also high in omega-3s. Most lamb is grass fed, and a half-pound portion will cost about four dollars at Whole Foods. Remember, as the quality of meat goes down, so does the price. For vegetarians and vegans, there are a whole host of replacement items you could use, which you already know about and love. Choose your favorite for this chili.

You should be able to get all these ingredients for about ten dollars, and this will serve several people with room for leftovers.

*1 onion (optional—there are some onions already in the
  store-bought salsa)*
Shaved fresh ginger (optional)
4 to 6 garlic cloves, smashed (optional)
Muchi Curry or other curry powder to taste (optional)
½ pound bison, lamb, or grass-fed beef
12 ounces salsa
2 15-ounce cans kidney beans (or fresh)
*½ pound chopped greens (Fresh spinach works great, but you can
  also use frozen greens here: spinach, kale, escarole, whatever you
  have.)*

If using extra onions, ginger, garlic, or curry, heat a little oil in your pot over medium heat, and then add the optional ingredients and sauté just until the onion starts to brown. This mix is a very powerful combination that has been shown to help fight all sorts of really nasty diseases.

Once the onion is browned, or if you are not using the optional ingredients, add your meat and the salsa, and mix together. Once it has started to cook, add the drained and rinsed beans. Mix it around. After 3 minutes, put the greens in, turn down the heat a touch and cover the pot. Let it simmer for a couple more minutes.

The greens cook almost instantly and the beans heat up quickly. The key is to make sure the meat thoroughly cooks.

Feel free to add more greens if you wish. You can serve this over quinoa or with other vegetables.

Orr's Island Vegetable Soup

Servings: 4   **Cheats/Serving: 0**

Our kitchen is seldom without a pot of vegetable soup made from whatever vegetables happen to look fresh in the market. My mother-in-law plays around with this recipe depending on what is available. You can add cooked garbanzos, white beans or any other kind of bean to make it a meal.

This soup is also perfect for your slow cooker. Cook it on high for about 4 hours or on low for 5 to 6 hours, depending on your cooker.

Some of the vegetables that go into the soup include chayote (pear-shaped pale green) and calabaza (dark green). Chayote (pronounced chai-o-tay), also known as the vegetable pear, mirliton, or christophene, is originally native to Mexico and Central America. Though mild and almost bland in taste, it is packed with nutrients and rich in amino acids and vitamin C. The leaves and fruit have diuretic, cardiovascular, and anti-inflammatory properties, and a tea made from the leaves has been used in the treatment of arteriosclerosis and hypertension, and to dissolve kidney stones.

8 cups of chicken broth
2 carrots, cut into chunks
1 onion, thickly sliced
4 to 5 garlic cloves, peeled and chopped
1 teaspoon chopped fresh ginger (optional)
Dash of turmeric powder (optional)
1 large tomato, cut into chunks

1 teaspoon minced jalapeño (more or less to your taste)
¼ pound calabaza squash, cut into chunks
1 chayote, cut into chunks
½ cabbage, roughly chopped
1 handful spinach, Swiss chard, or other leafy green
Juice of 1 lime or ½ lemon
Fresh cilantro, chopped

In a large stockpot, bring the broth to a boil.

Add the carrots, onion, garlic, ginger, turmeric, and tomato, and simmer over medium heat for 6 to 7 minutes.

Add the jalapeño, calabaza, and chayote, and simmer until the vegetables are almost cooked. Add the cabbage and leafy greens, and cook for another few minutes.

Turn off the heat and add the lime or lemon juice. Garnish with cilantro.

PEERtrainer Cleanse Soup

Servings: 10   **Cheats/Serving: 1**

1 teaspoon coconut or olive oil
1 large yellow or sweet onion, chopped
1½ pounds white button mushrooms, sliced
32 ounces chicken or mushroom broth
One 13.5-ounce can unsweetened coconut milk
2 large heads broccoli, chopped
1 large head cauliflower, chopped
1 pound spinach (optional)
2 fingers' worth of fresh ginger, peeled
1 finger's worth of fresh turmeric, peeled
5 garlic cloves, crushed
Sea salt to taste

Heat a stockpot over medium heat. Add the oil, and once it's warm, add the onion to the pot.

Brown the onions while stirring constantly. Once they're light brown, add the mushrooms and continue to cook until the mushrooms are light brown.

Add the broth and coconut milk, and then turn the heat up to high.

Add the broccoli, cauliflower, spinach, ginger, turmeric, and garlic, and bring to a boil. Turn the heat down and simmer for 15 minutes.

Let the soup stand for 10 minutes before using an immersion blender to blend it until smooth. Taste and add salt as needed.

Spicy Pumpkin Ginger Soup

Servings: 10 to 12   **Cheats/Serving: 1**

This soup is a Thanksgiving staple in our home. Served by the fireside as a first course, it never fails to wow guests. That said, there's no reason you couldn't serve it chilled in the summertime as well.

2 tablespoons olive oil
2 cups finely chopped onion
2 garlic cloves, minced
1 small potato, boiled, peeled, and cubed
1½ tablespoons ginger, minced
⅛ teaspoon ground cardamom
¼ teaspoon freshly grated nutmeg
1 tablespoon curry powder
¾ teaspoon cayenne pepper (or more to taste)
4 cups chicken or vegetable broth
Salt to taste
Two 15-ounce cans solid-pack pumpkin

2 cups water
One 13.5-ounce can unsweetened coconut milk
2 tablespoons cilantro, chopped
1 jalapeño, minced
Juice of ½ lemon

In a large stockpot over medium heat, add the olive oil. Once it's hot, add the onion. Cook, stirring occasionally, until softened, about 5 minutes. Add the garlic, potato, and minced ginger, and continue cooking for 1 minute, stirring constantly.

Add the spices and 2 cups broth, and then purée using an immersion blender and a little broth.

Add the salt, pumpkin, water, the remaining broth, and coconut milk, stirring to combine, and simmer gently, uncovered, about 20 minutes.

Add cilantro, jalapeño, and lemon. Puree one more time and serve.

Serve immediately.

TNT's Veggie Weight-Loss Soup

Servings: 12   **Cheats/Serving: 0.5**

This recipe is from someone who did not like my soup, so she made her own! It's best when it's served piping hot. The possibilities for this soup are endless—leave out vegetables you don't like or add in those you do. Substitute brown rice or quinoa for the lentils, or top with crumbled oyster crackers or saltines.

One 16-ounce bag of lentils
2 to 3 zucchinis, sliced and quartered, about 4 cups
One 8-ounce package sliced baby bella mushrooms, about 3 cups
6 celery stalks, sliced, about 2 cups
Garlic powder to taste
Two 48-ounce cans chicken or vegetable broth, divided
Two 15-ounce cans stir-fry vegetables, drained
One 10-ounce box frozen chopped spinach
One 16-ounce bag frozen crinkle cut carrots
One 16-ounce bag frozen cut green beans
One 14-ounce bag frozen baby broccoli florets
Cayenne pepper to taste

Cook the lentils according to package directions (usually 1 part lentils to 1 part water).

In a large stockpot, combine zucchini, mushrooms, and celery. Sprinkle with garlic powder, stir, and add a cup or so of broth. Cook over high heat until the zucchini and celery start to become translucent. Be careful not to overcook the vegetables.

Turn the burner off, but leave the pot on the stove. Add the stir-fry vegetables.

One by one, microwave the frozen vegetables (per individual cooking instructions) and then add them to the stockpot.

Add all the remaining broth and the cooked lentils. Stir gently with a big spoon. Sprinkle with cayenne pepper and stir again.

Warm Applewood Bacon Soup

Servings: 4   **Cheats/Serving: .5**

This is one of our most popular soups!

2 slices applewood bacon
3 medium garlic cloves, minced or pressed
1 medium sweet onion, thinly sliced into 2-inch-long strips
1 head cauliflower, chopped into 2-inch pieces
32 ounces chicken broth
1 teaspoon rosemary, finely chopped
½ pound fresh spinach leaves
1 to 2 squeezes of fresh lemon juice
Sea salt and freshly ground pepper to taste

In a large 12- or 16-ounce skillet, cook the bacon over medium-low heat until it's crisp. Use tongs to take out the bacon and place it on doubled paper towels. Drain most of bacon grease, leaving just a little to cook the rest of the ingredients in.

Add garlic, onion, and cauliflower to the skillet over medium heat, and stir until the cauliflower and onion start to turn golden brown. Add the chicken broth, rosemary, and spinach, and cook until the cauliflower and spinach are tender, anywhere from 5 to 10 minutes.

Remove from heat. Stir in the bacon and add the lemon juice, salt, and pepper to desired taste.

Warm Cream of Tomato Soup

Servings: 8   **Cheats/Serving: 1**

One 13.5-ounce can unsweetened coconut milk
3 pounds canned tomatoes
3 garlic cloves, minced
Salt and pepper to taste

Place a pot over high heat. Add all the ingredients and bring to a boil. Once the soup is boiling, turn the heat down and let it simmer just a minute or two.

With an immersion blender, blend the soup until smooth.

Weight-Loss Shortcut Soup

Servings: 8   **Cheats/Serving: 1**

This soup travels wonderfully in a Thermos. Try it with the Italian Herb Goddess Chicken on page 255.

3 large heads broccoli (including stems)
5 garlic cloves
1 box (32 ounces) organic chicken, mushroom, or vegetable broth
One 13.5-ounce can unsweetened coconut milk
½ pound fresh spinach leaves
½ jalapeño, chopped (optional)
Sea salt and pepper to taste (optional)

Cut the broccoli into quarters and mince the garlic.

Place the broth, coconut milk, broccoli, spinach, garlic, jalapeño, salt, and pepper in a large stockpot over high heat.

When the mixture begins to boil, turn down the heat and simmer for 20 minutes.

With an immersion blender, blend the soup until it's smooth. Taste, and add more salt and pepper if needed.

SLOW COOKER AND STEWS

Classic Pork Loin Roast Tacos

Servings: 12   **Cheats/Serving: 2**

3 pounds boneless pork loin roast, cubed
½ teaspoon sea salt
Two 4-ounce cans diced green chili peppers
3 garlic cloves, minced
1½ cups water
¼ cup chipotle sauce
1 head of lettuce, quartered

Place the pork in a slow cooker and cover with salt, peppers, and garlic, and then pour the water and the chipotle sauce on top.

Cover and cook on low for 6 hours.

Remove the pork from the slow cooker, and with 2 forks, shred the pork.

Return the meat to the slow cooker and allow it to sit in the juices for 15 minutes.

Serve wrapped in lettuce.

Dad's Hearty Beef Stew

Servings: 8   **Cheats/Serving: 3**

2 pounds organic beef stew meat, cut into 1-inch chunks
2 cups carrots, chopped
1 cup celery, chopped
3 medium onions, chopped
5 tablespoons olive oil
5 tablespoons almond flour or almond meal
One 15-ounce can tomato sauce
1 cup low-sodium beef broth

Add all the ingredients to a slow cooker. Cook on medium heat 4 to 6 hours, or until the beef is tender.

New Orleans Chicken and Sausage Gumbo

Servings: 6   **Cheats/Serving: 1**

Try this over brown cauliflower rice (recipe page 273) or steamed broccoli.

¾ cup boneless, skinless free-range chicken breasts, cubed
¼ pound cooked, smoked sausage, chopped
2 celery stalks with leaves, sliced
1 large carrot, chopped
1 medium onion
One 14½–ounce can stewed tomatoes
5 cups water
1 teaspoon thyme
One 10-ounce package frozen, cut okra, thawed and drained

Mix all the ingredients except the okra into a slow cooker. Cover and cook on low heat for 6½ to 7 hours.

Stir in the okra and cook for 20 more minutes.

Slow-Cooker Chicken and Spinach Soup

Servings: 4   **Cheats/Serving: 2**

Leftovers of roasted chicken work best in this recipe, though cooked breast pieces will work, too

1 pound chicken, cut into bite-sized pieces
1 pound fresh spinach
2 yellow onions, diced
2 teaspoons of red pepper flakes (optional)
Salt and pepper to taste
32 ounces organic chicken broth

In a slow cooker, add all the ingredients and stir. Simmer on low heat for 3 hours. Watch while it's cooking in case more broth or water is needed. Adjust seasonings before serving.

Slow-Cooker Clean-Eating Cheat-Free Soup

Servings: 4   **Cheats/Serving: 0**

1 carrot, chopped
1 large onion, chopped
1 tablespoon olive oil
One 14½-ounce can organic stewed tomatoes
2 cups chopped cabbage
1 teaspoon sea salt
¼ teaspoon pepper
⅔ cup dried lima beans
¼ cup parsley, chopped
2 cups water or unsweetened coconut water

Add all the ingredients to a slow cooker. Cook on medium heat for 3 to 4 hours, or until the beans are soft.

Slow-Cooker Fire-Roasted Tomato Beef Chili

Servings: 8   **Cheats/Serving: 2**

2 pounds beef stew meat, cut into 1-inch chunks
1 large yellow onion, diced
8 ounces fresh mushrooms, sliced
2 medium carrots, chopped
2 tablespoons chili powder
1 teaspoon cumin
1 teaspoon garlic salt
One 28-ounce can diced tomatoes
One 28-ounce can fire-roasted tomatoes
1/2 teaspoon oregano
1 tablespoon olive or coconut oil
28 ounces water
2 teaspoons sea salt (optional)

Add all the ingredients to a slow cooker. Cook on medium heat for 4 to 6 hours, until the beef is thoroughly cooked.

Slow-Cooker Garlic and Herb Roasted Chicken

Servings: 16 to 20   **Cheats/Serving: 2**

This recipe works best with a chicken that has a pop-up timer.

4- to 5-pound roasting chicken
1/2 cup coconut oil
2 teaspoons paprika
4 garlic gloves, minced
Salt and pepper to taste

Prep the chicken by cleaning out the cavity so no innards are left. Rub hardened coconut oil all over the chicken, and then rub paprika, garlic, salt, and pepper all over the chicken, both inside and out.

Place the chicken in a slow cooker. Cook on high for 1 hour, and then reduce the heat to low and cook an additional 5 hours until the meat is tender.

Slow-Cooker Wraps

Servings: varies   **Cheats/Serving: varies based on the protein**

Leftover protein or casserole from the slow cooker
Large cabbage leaves

Add leftovers to the large cabbage leaves, wrapping the leaf around the leftovers. If you want to transport this, wrap tinfoil around the cabbage leaf.

OVEN BAKED AND CASSEROLES

Brian's Sweet Potato and Coconut Meatballs

Servings: 4 (4 to 6 meatballs)   **Cheats/Serving: 2**

Brian Rigby is a performance nutrition expert who is not only a writer at PEERtrainer but also runs a thriving practice in Boulder.

Brian says, "When I can find 95 percent lean, grass-fed ground beef on sale, I'll make up some meatballs (or hamburgers, depending on my whim). I tend to be a little random in what I put into them, but here's a recipe I'll use from time to time. The sweet potato keeps the meatballs moist, which is useful because the extra-lean beef doesn't have a lot of fat!"

1 pound 95 percent lean grass-fed ground beef
1 cup sweet potato, grated
½ cup unsweetened shredded coconut
*4 to 8 garlic cloves, minced (I love garlic, but not everybody is as in
    love with it as I am . . . use less if you want less!)*
1 teaspoon black pepper
Cayenne pepper to taste
Salt to taste

Preheat oven to 400 degrees F. Line a baking sheet with parchment paper.

Mix the beef, sweet potato, coconut, garlic, black pepper, cayenne pepper, and salt in a bowl. Form meatballs 1 to 1½ inches in diameter and place on the lined baking sheet.

Bake 30 to 35 minutes, or until browned on the outside and no longer pink on the inside.

These can be served any way you'd normally serve meatballs, or you can toss them in a soup or on a salad for an easy protein option.

Chicken Bake

Servings: 8   **Cheats/Serving: 1.5**

4 boneless, skinless free-range chicken breasts
Salt and pepper to taste
1 tablespoon olive oil
4 medium carrots, thinly sliced
2 medium zucchini, thinly sliced
12 mushrooms, thinly sliced
4 green onion, thinly sliced
2 thumbs' worth of ginger, minced
4 tablespoons tamari

Preheat oven to 400 degrees F.

Cut 4 pieces of parchment paper, each large enough to wrap a chicken breast and ¼ of the vegetables. Coat the chicken breasts with salt and pepper. Place one breast on each piece of parchment paper.

Drizzle olive oil over each chicken breast. Add ¼ of the vegetables and ginger and 1 tablespoon of tamari to each packet. Loosely wrap each chicken breast and vegetable mixture with the parchment paper.

Place the packets on a baking sheet and bake 30 to 35 minutes, or until the chicken is thoroughly cooked (there should be no pink left when the chicken is cut open).

Chicken, Artichoke, Mushroom, with Parmesan Casserole

Servings: 8   **Cheats/Serving: 2**

This mushroom mixture is a great addition to any traditional protein like grilled chicken, or atop a bed of mixed greens.

2 pounds chicken breast

Mushroom Mixture
1 8-ounce box or bag mushrooms
½ pound cherry tomatoes
6 garlic cloves
8 tablespoons cilantro
½ pound artichoke hearts, quartered and rinsed
4 tablespoons olive oil
Juice of ½ lemon
Salt and pepper to taste
1 to 2 teaspoons red pepper flakes (or more to taste)
1 pound spinach
Goat cheese or Parmesan confetti (optional)

Preheat oven to 350 degrees F.

Heat a frying pan over medium heat. Once hot, brown the chicken breast on all sides.

While the chicken is browning, prepare the mushroom mixture. Slice the mushrooms into small pieces, about 4 to 5 per mushroom. Slice the cherry tomatoes in half. Crush the garlic cloves and chop the cilantro leaves, throwing the stems away.

In a large mixing bowl, mix the mushrooms, tomatoes, garlic, cilantro, artichoke hearts, olive oil, and lemon juice. Add the salt, pepper, and red pepper flakes.

In a casserole dish, evenly distribute the spinach around the bottom and then place in the browned chicken breast. Add the mushroom mixture on top of the chicken, and top with goat cheese or Parmesan confetti.

Bake for 30 minutes.

Coconut Chicken Tenders

Servings: 3   **Cheats/Serving: 3**

Serve these chicken tenders with fresh vegetables.

¼ cup walnuts
¼ cup almonds
7 tablespoons shredded unsweetened coconut
⅛ teaspoon garlic powder
⅛ teaspoon pepper
⅛ teaspoon salt
⅓ cup egg substitute or 3 egg whites
6 (about 12 ounces) free-range chicken tenderloins

Preheat oven to 375 degrees F.

In a food processor, grind the walnuts and almonds. Add the ground nuts to a bowl and mix in the coconut flakes, garlic powder, and pepper and salt.

Whisk the egg substitute in a separate bowl.

Coat a baking dish with nonstick cooking spray or line the dish with parchment paper.

Dip the chicken into the eggs and then into the coconut mixture. Place the chicken in the baking dish.

Bake for 25 to 30 minutes, turning once, halfway through. The chicken is done when it is no longer pink in the center and the coconut is golden brown.

Cold Winter's Night Casserole

Servings: 8   **Cheats/Serving: 2**

2½ pounds eggplant
1 teaspoon salt, plus some for sprinkling on the eggplant
1 to 2 onions, diced
2 tablespoons olive oil
1 potato, thinly sliced
1 pound ground lamb
½ teaspoon black pepper
⅛ cup of red wine
⅛ cup chicken broth
¼ teaspoon red pepper flakes
1 teaspoon cinnamon
1 tomato, chopped
1 small can of tomato sauce
3 tablespoons chopped parsley
½ cup water
Parmesan cheese

Topping
1 tablespoon butter
1 tablespoon olive oil
2 tablespoons flour
2 cups unsweetened coconut milk (So Delicious is our preferred brand)
¼ teaspoon of salt
⅛ teaspoon white pepper
4 to 5 grates of fresh nutmeg

Preheat oven to 375 degrees F.

Slice the eggplant thinly. Sprinkle with salt and allow the juices to drain away in a colander for 30 minutes. Squeeze the juices out, rinse with cold water, and pat dry. Fry each slice lightly in a non-stick pan.

Fry the onion in the olive oil until golden. Add the potato and fry for a few minutes. Add the ground lamb, salt, and pepper, and fry until brown. Add the red wine and let it reduce some. Then add the chicken broth and red pepper flakes. Add the cinnamon, tomato and tomato sauce, parsley, and water. Simmer 15 minutes until the water is absorbed.

Alternate the layers of eggplant slices and meat/onion mixture in a 9-by-11 casserole dish. Top every other layer with a sprinkling of Parmesan cheese.

To make the topping, melt the butter in the saucepan and add the olive oil. Add the flour and stir over a low heat for a few minutes until well blended. When the flour smells slightly nutty, add the coconut milk gradually, stirring until it boils. Use a whisk so lumps do not form. Season with salt, white pepper, and fresh nutmeg. Simmer until the sauce thickens. Pour the sauce over the eggplant and meat mixture and bake, uncovered, for 45 minutes. Cut into squares to serve.

Favorite Roast Chicken

Servings: 8   **Cheats/Serving: 2**

Tip: Make this chicken on a beer-can chicken roaster. You can buy one at Crate and Barrel, Williams-Sonoma, Amazon.com, or World Market. They are inexpensive and can be used for any chicken dish you cook.

2 teaspoons hot Hungarian paprika
2 teaspoons onion powder

2 teaspoons garlic powder
1 tablespoon olive oil
1 teaspoon salt
1 teaspoon pepper
1 whole roasting chicken

Preheat oven to 400 degrees F.

Mix together the spices, oil, salt, and pepper.

Rinse the chicken and pat it dry with paper towels. Slather the spice mixture all over the chicken.

Place the chicken in a roasting pan and roast for 1 hour and 45 minutes.

Let it rest for 20 minutes before eating so all the juices go back into the bird.

Hearty Meatloaf Muffins

Servings: 8   **Cheats/Serving: 2**

This recipe makes a lot of servings, but they freeze well to eat later!

2 pounds ground grass-fed beef
2 red onions, finely chopped
4 garlic cloves, minced
½ red pepper, finely chopped
½ cup cilantro, chopped
½ cup parsley, chopped
2 teaspoons cumin
1 teaspoon pepper
3 omega 3–enriched eggs

Preheat oven to 400 degrees F.

Add all the ingredients to a resealable food storage bag, and mash together until it's well mixed.

Scoop out the mixture into muffin tins, then bake for 45 minutes.

Hot Italian Salmon Garlic Scampi

Servings: 4   **Cheats/Serving: 2**

People say that this tastes like shrimp scampi but without the pasta and shrimp! With six ingredients and six minutes of prep time, make a dish I've never had anyone dislike.

Fresh salmon is the key to this recipe. If it isn't fresh, it just doesn't taste as good.

Juice of 1 lemon
1 pound fresh salmon
1½ tablespoons olive oil
7 garlic cloves, fresh and crushed (enough to cover the salmon completely!)
10 shakes red pepper flakes
4 shakes salt

Preheat oven to 400 degrees F.

In a large casserole dish, place a large piece of tinfoil large enough to wrap completely around the salmon. Squeeze a bit of fresh lemon juice on the tinfoil so the salmon doesn't stick.

Place salmon in the pan and drizzle olive oil on top. Then squeeze remaining lemon juice over the fish. Add garlic, red pepper flakes, and salt, being sure to spread everything evenly over the salmon. Seal the tinfoil.

Place in the oven for 28 minutes, and then use a knife to check. The fish should flake easily. It will most likely need 5 to 10 minutes more (33 to 38 minutes total), depending on your oven. Try not to overcook the fish.

Any leftover salmon makes a great protein for other meals.

Italian Herb Goddess Chicken

Servings: 1   **Cheats/Serving: 1.5**

Serve this chicken with the Cream of Broccoli Weight-Loss CheatCut Soup on page 229.

*1 organic, boneless, skinless chicken breast
   (4 ounces)
1 teaspoon oil
Salt and pepper to taste
1 lemon, sliced
1 lime, sliced
1 handful fresh herbs (basil and oregano are favorites)*

Preheat oven to 350 degrees F.

Rub the chicken breast with oil, salt, and pepper. In a baking dish, place a piece of tinfoil large enough to wrap the chicken.

Place the chicken on the foil, then lay the lemon and lime slices on top of the chicken. Rinse the fresh herbs and lay them on top of lemon and lime. Fold the tinfoil over the chicken and seal the edges.

Bake for 25 to 35 minutes.

Japanese Chili Salmon

Servings: 4   **Cheats/Serving: 2**

This salmon makes great leftovers to accompany other meals.

1 pound fresh salmon
1 tablespoon olive oil
1 teaspoon fresh sesame seeds
4 shakes red pepper flakes or 1 shake cayenne pepper
4 shakes salt

Preheat oven to 400 degrees F.

In a large casserole dish, place a piece of tinfoil large enough to wrap the salmon.

Place the salmon on the tinfoil and drizzle with the olive oil. Add the sesame seeds, red pepper flakes or cayenne pepper, and salt, being sure to spread everything evenly over the salmon. Seal the tinfoil around the salmon.

Bake for 25 minutes.

Lemon Herb Salmon

Servings: 4   **Cheats/Serving: 2**

2 fresh lemons
½ tablespoon olive oil
1 garlic clove, minced
Salt and pepper to taste
1 pound salmon fillets
1 cup fresh dill, chopped

Preheat oven to 450 degrees F. Line a baking sheet with tinfoil or parchment paper, big enough to wrap the salmon.

Cut one lemon in slices and one lemon in quarters (to get the juice). Combine olive oil, garlic, and lemon juice from the quartered lemon in a small bowl with salt and pepper.

Spread the mixture evenly over the fish. Place the fish skin side down on the foil or parchment paper. Sprinkle the chopped dill all over and around the fish (use all your dill!) and then top with the lemon slices. Close the parchment paper or foil so salmon is inside.

Cook for 10 minutes or until salmon flakes with a fork. You can serve with more lemon slices if you want.

Mint and Shallot Halibut with Kale and Oven-Roasted Tomatoes

Servings: 4   **Cheats/Serving: 1.5**

1 pound tomatoes
1 tablespoon olive oil
1 pound halibut
2 mint sprigs
5 tablespoons shallot, minced
1 pound kale
½ cup vegetable broth

Preheat oven to 450 degrees F.

Depending on the size of your tomatoes, either roughly chop them or halve them. Spread the tomatoes out evenly on a baking sheet, and then drizzle with the olive oil. Bake for 25 to 30 minutes.

While the tomatoes are baking, place a piece of tinfoil large enough to wrap the fish into an oven-safe baking dish. Add the halibut to the middle of the foil, and then evenly distribute the mint and shallot over the fish. Wrap the foil tightly around the fish. When the tomatoes have about 10 minutes left, add the fish to the oven. Everything should be done about the same time—just make sure the fish is opaque.

Remove the stems from the kale, and then roughly chop the leaves. In a large saucepan over medium heat, add the vegetable broth. Once the broth is simmering, add the kale and cook until it's wilted.

To serve, add the kale to the bottom of your dish and then place the tomatoes on top. Add the halibut on top of your bed of kale and tomatoes.

Poisson en Papillote

Servings: 8   **Cheats/Serving: 1.5 per 4-ounce serving**

1/2 cup freshly squeezed lemon juice
1/2 teaspoon sea salt
1/4 onion, minced
3 garlic cloves, minced
1/8 teaspoon paprika
1/8 teaspoon pepper
Four 8-ounce wild-caught Alaskan salmon fillets
1 fresh lemon, quartered

Add all the ingredients except the salmon and lemon quarters to a resealable food storage bag. Seal the bag and shake to mix.

Add the salmon to the bag and shake it to make sure each fillet is well coated. Refrigerate overnight, turning occasionally.

Preheat oven to 450 degrees F.

Cut 8 sheets of parchment paper, each measuring 12 inches by 17 inches (each fillet gets 2 sheets). Fold each one in half crosswise, then open and lay them flat.

Remove the salmon from the bag and discard the remaining marinade. Lay each fillet on one side of the parchment paper. Fold the paper over the salmon, making small, overlapping pleats as you go along to create a half-moon shape. Place the packets on a baking dish.

Bake for 8 minutes. Serve with a lemon wedge.

Sesame and Honey Chicken

Servings: 8   **Cheats/Serving: 3**

Serve this chicken with Cheat-Free Stir-Fry or Cauliflower Rice.

1 cup pure raw unfiltered honey
6 tablespoons organic tamari
4 boneless, skinless free-range chicken breasts
½ cup sesame seeds

Preheat oven to 350 degrees F.

In a resealable food storage bag, add the honey, tamari, and chicken. Mix well, completely coating the chicken.

Remove the chicken from the bag and bake on a baking sheet for 10 minutes.

Meanwhile, add the sesame seeds to a mixing bowl. Remove the chicken from the oven and coat well with the sesame seeds.

Return the chicken to the oven for 10 more minutes, or until the chicken is no longer pink in the center.

Shepherd's Pie

Servings: 10   **Cheats/Serving: 3**

4 tablespoons olive oil, divided
1 large onion, chopped
1 pound grass-fed or nitrate-free bacon or turkey bacon, chopped
2 medium carrots, diced
2 celery stalks, diced
1 pound grass-fed ground beef
½ teaspoon sea salt
1 teaspoon freshly ground pepper
1 cup organic or homemade chicken broth
2 large heads cauliflower, chopped

Heat 2 tablespoons of the olive oil in a large frying pan over medium heat. Sauté the onion until it's soft and browned, about 15 minutes.

Add the bacon and cook for 10 minutes. Add the carrots and celery, and then cook an additional 10 minutes.

Add the ground beef and cook until it's brown. Mix in the salt and pepper, and then add the chicken broth and bring it to a simmer, cooking until the broth is about 60 percent evaporated.

Meanwhile, preheat oven to 350 degrees F.

Bring 1 to 2 inches of water to boil in a stockpot. Place the cauliflower in the stockpot or place it in a steamer basket in the stockpot. Cover and cook until the cauliflower is soft, about 10 minutes.

Drain the cauliflower and add it to a food processor or blender. Add the remaining 2 tablespoons of olive oil and process until smooth.

Pour the beef mixture into a baking dish and then layer the cauliflower on top. Sprinkle with extra bacon bits if desired.

Bake for 30 minutes.

Protein Based (tradition and lean)

Arroz Con Pollo

Servings: 4   **Cheats/Serving: 2**

3 bell peppers (as many different colors as you can)
2 small yellow onions
1 cup broccoli (sounds strange but is delicious!)
1 pound chicken breast, cut into bite-sized pieces
Cayenne pepper to taste
Adobo seasoning to taste
$\frac{1}{2}$ tablespoon olive oil
2 garlic cloves, chopped
Chopped jalapeños to taste (optional)
$\frac{1}{2}$ cup green olives (optional)
$\frac{1}{2}$ cup chicken broth
1 cup water
$\frac{1}{2}$ cup cooked rice (Mexican rice is best)
Dried cilantro to taste
Dried parsley to taste

Dice the bell peppers, onions, and broccoli. Coat the chicken breasts in cayenne pepper and adobo. Word to the wise: less cayenne pepper is more for those who don't like it hot; you can never put too much adobo on chicken.

Put a large saucepan (that you have a cover for) on the stove over medium heat.

When the pan is hot, add the olive oil. Once that's hot, add the garlic, onions, and jalapeños. Cook these until onions are almost translucent, about 3 minutes. Add the chicken breast. Cook until outsides are not pink but the chicken is not fully cooked, about 3 minutes. Add olives if you are using them (a little of the juice from the jar is also delicious in this recipe). Add chicken broth and let simmer for 2 to 3 minutes. Add vegetables and water, and then cover so that the mixture can steam. Check every 5 minutes to see if you need to add more water.

Cover until vegetables are soft but not fully cooked; add rice and remove cover. Add in herbs. When the water has evaporated and chicken is fully cooked, this is ready to serve.

Cheat-Free Stir-Fry

Servings: 6   **Cheats/Serving: 1**

If you don't have a leek, feel free to use an onion in this recipe. This can be combined with rice or quinoa.

1 tablespoon olive oil
2 garlic cloves, minced
1 leek, chopped (you can use an onion instead of leeks)
1 pound chicken or grass-fed beef, cut into strips
1 head broccoli, chopped into bite-sized pieces/individual florets
1 red pepper, sliced
One 16-ounce package snow peas
One 8-ounce can sliced water chestnuts
Fresh ginger, peeled and chopped, to taste
½ tablespoon soy sauce

Add the olive oil to a wok and heat over medium heat. When oil is hot, add 1 garlic clove and the leek. When the leek is translucent, remove from the pan and set aside, leaving the oil in the pan.

Add chicken or beef and the other garlic clove. Cook until the outside of the protein is done. Add the vegetables and stir-fry until they are cooked. (If the oil evaporates, feel free to use water.) When the vegetables and protein are cooked, add in the leek, ginger, and soy sauce. When the leek and ginger have heated, remove and serve.

Chicken Marsala

Servings: 8   **Cheats/Serving: 2**

⅓ cup almond flour, divided
1 teaspoon minced garlic
1 teaspoon minced onions
1 teaspoon coarse sea salt
½ teaspoon coarsely ground black pepper
4 boneless, skinless free-range chicken breasts, cut in half lengthwise
2 tablespoons extra virgin olive or coconut oil
8 ounces mushrooms, sliced
½ cup organic low-sodium chicken broth or homemade stock
¾ cup Marsala wine
1 tablespoon grass-fed butter
1 teaspoon basil leaves
¾ teaspoon parsley flakes for garnish

Add all but 1 tablespoon of the flour into a resealable food storage bag. Add the garlic, onion, salt, and pepper. Seal the bag and shake to mix.

Add the chicken breasts to the bag, seal, and shake to coat them thoroughly with the flour mixture.

In a large skillet over medium-high heat, heat the olive oil. When it's hot, cook several pieces of chicken 3 minutes per side, or until they are golden brown and no longer pink in the center. Remove the chicken from the skillet and keep it warm under a dish or tinfoil. Repeat until all the chicken is cooked.

Add the mushrooms to the same skillet and cook until tender, about 5 minutes.

Meanwhile, mix the broth and the reserved tablespoon of flour in a bowl. Add the mixture to the skillet. Slowly stir in the wine. Bring this mixture to a boil, stirring to release the browned bits on the bottom of the skillet.

Stir the butter and basil into the skillet, cooking 2 more minutes, or until the sauce thickens.

Place the chicken on a serving dish, cover with the mushroom sauce, and garnish with parsley flakes.

Chickpea and Spinach Curry with Cucumber-Avocado Sauce

Servings: 4   Cheats/Serving: 1

1 tablespoon coconut oil
1 large sweet onion, chopped
2 tablespoons curry powder
4 garlic cloves, chopped
1 tablespoon fresh ginger, chopped
2 cups plus 1 teaspoon water, divided
Two 15.5-ounce cans chickpeas, or 2 pounds fresh chickpeas
1½ pounds spinach, chopped
1 cucumber, seeded and chopped
1 avocado, chopped
Juice of 1 lime
¼ cup cilantro
Sea salt to taste
Large bowl of mixed greens
Lime wedges for garnish

Heat the oil in a large saucepan over medium heat. Add the onion and sauté until very light brown. Be sure to watch the onion so it doesn't burn.

Add the curry powder, garlic, ginger, and 1 teaspoon of water to the pan and cook for 30 seconds.

Add the chickpeas, spinach, and 2 cups of water to the saucepan. Bring to a simmer and cook until the mixture is slightly thickened, about 10 minutes.

While the chickpea mixture is cooking, put the cucumber, avocado, lime juice, cilantro, and salt in a blender and blend until smooth.

Serve the chickpea mixture on a bed of mixed greens, topped with the sauce. Add lime wedges for garnish.

Ginger Salmon with Bok Choy and Spinach

Servings: 4   **Cheats/Serving: 2**

1 tablespoon olive or coconut oil, divided
1 pound skinless salmon filet, sliced into 4 equal pieces
Sea salt
¼ cup plus 1 teaspoon water, divided
4 scallions, thinly sliced
2 garlic cloves, chopped
1 tablespoon ginger, chopped
1 pound spinach
1 pound baby bok choy, halved lengthwise
Juice of 1 lime
1 teaspoon cilantro (optional)
Red pepper flakes to taste (optional)

Heat ½ tablespoon of the oil in a large skillet over medium-high heat.

Season the salmon with salt and then cook in the skillet, approximately 4 to 5 minutes per side.

In a separate skillet over medium-high heat, add the remaining ½ tablespoon of oil and 1 teaspoon of water. Add the scallions, garlic, and ginger, and stir continuously for 30 seconds.

Add the spinach, bok choy, and ¼ cup of water. Stir continuously for 4 to 6 minutes, or until the vegetables are bright green.

Place the salmon and vegetables on a plate and squeeze the lime juice over the top. Garnish with cilantro and red pepper flakes, if desired.

Grilled Lemon and Tamari Shrimp with Basil

Servings: 5   **Cheats/Serving: 3**

1 cup fresh lemon juice
2 tablespoons tamari
4 teaspoons seafood seasoning
2 teaspoons lemon pepper
1 teaspoon dried basil
4 garlic cloves, minced
1/2 cup olive oil
1 pound medium raw shrimp, peeled and deveined

Add all the ingredients except the shrimp to a large resealable food storage bag. Mix well and then add the shrimp, making sure they are entirely covered. Refrigerate the shrimp for at least 30 minutes.

Preheat oven to 400 degrees F, or heat the grill to medium heat.

Cut a piece of tinfoil large enough so that all the shrimp will lay on top. Place the shrimp on the foil on either the oven rack or the grill. Cut a second piece of tinfoil the same size and place it over the top of the shrimp, crimping all the edges. Make a slit in the top and then cook for 6 minutes.

Mix before serving.

Honey Ginger Dijon Marinated Chicken Breasts

Servings: 8 to 12   **Cheats/Serving: 2**

1/2 cup organic tamari
1/2 cup pineapple juice

¼ cup olive oil
1 teaspoon dry mustard
1 tablespoon pure unfiltered raw honey
1 teaspoon ground ginger
1 teaspoon garlic
½ teaspoon freshly ground black pepper
4 to 6 boneless, skinless free-range chicken breasts

Combine all the ingredients except the chicken in a 1-gallon resealable food storage bag and mix well.

Add the chicken to the bag and refrigerate for 24 hours.

Grill the chicken until it is no longer pink in the center.

Mussels with Coconut Curry Sauce

Servings: 14   **Cheats/Serving: 2**

This is the best coconut curry sauce recipe out there for mussels. There are subtle differences in this recipe that make it better than anything you'll see on the Internet or even in gourmet restaurants. We make this claim after eating Sukanya Wicks's recipe and also trying a disappointing version at a well-respected Colorado restaurant.

This sauce can also be used for almost any seafood. It also makes an excellent replacement for butter (try it with lobster!). You can also cook shrimp, scallops, cod, halibut, and even salmon using this recipe.

Unlike other recipes we publish at PEERtrainer, this one needs to be followed as closely as possible to achieve the precise flavor. A hint here is that the combination of cilantro, lime, and scallion will make or break this recipe. You want to make sure you have enough of this combination to bring out the flavor, but you don't want any single ingredient to overpower the others.

This is a great general rule of thumb when cooking with spices. Many people who are new to using spices tend to overdo it. While that is fine when you start, know that balance is the goal and is what separates average cooks from great ones.

5 pounds mussels (preferably cultivated), scrubbed and rinsed
A little olive oil
1½ tablespoons minced garlic
1 tablespoon minced ginger (or more to taste)
½ tablespoon Thai red curry paste (or more to taste)
⅓ cup dry white wine (optional)
1 tablespoon sugar
One 13.5-ounce can unsweetened coconut milk
2 cups fresh cilantro
About 3 scallions, thinly sliced
Juice of 3 limes
1 tablespoon slivered ginger
Lime wedges for garnish

Scrub mussels well and remove the beards. Cultivated mussels just need a good rinse.

Heat a pan over medium-low heat. Add a tiny amount of olive oil, and then sauté garlic and ginger for about 10 seconds.

Add the curry paste, white wine, sugar, and coconut milk. Cook over high heat for about 2 minutes.

Add the mussels and cilantro (saving some cilantro for garnish) and toss well. Cook mussels covered for 5 to 8 minutes. Shake the pot a few times, and then discard any unopened mussels.

Garnish with more cilantro, scallions, lime juice, and slivered ginger. Serve with lime wedges.

Shrimp Taco Wraps with Black Beans

Servings: 4   **Cheats/Serving: 1.5**

Swap the shrimp for chicken for a variation on this recipe. The chicken should be seasoned with salt and cooked through, about 6 to 7 minutes on a side in a skillet over medium heat.

1 tablespoon olive oil, divided
1 pound deveined shrimp
Kosher salt to taste
4 scallions, sliced, white and green parts separated
One 15.5-ounce can black beans, rinsed, or 1 pound fresh
    black beans
1/4 cup water
1/2 avocado
Salsa
Cilantro, chopped
4 lime wedges
1 large head of cabbage, leaves separated

In a large skillet over medium heat, heat 1/2 tablespoon olive oil.

Season the shrimp with a little salt and cook in the skillet until cooked through, usually 3 to 5 minutes on each side, until they're opaque and pink or orange.

In a separate pan, heat the remaining olive oil over medium heat. Add the white parts of the scallions, stirring until soft, 1 to 2 minutes. Add the beans, water, and a shake of salt. Cook until warmed, about 4 minutes.

Stir in the green parts of the scallions.

To serve, place the bean mixture, shrimp, chopped avocado, salsa, cilantro, and lime wedges in small bowls. Place the cabbage leaves on the table as wraps, and everyone can make their own.

Spicy Thai Curry

Servings: 8   **Cheats/Serving: 1 + (2 per ½ cup rice)**

This curry is a gift that keeps on giving—make a huge pot and eat it over the next three days. It tastes better every time you reheat!

Curry is extremely customizable. Add whatever vegetables you like or have on hand, and while I like basmati rice, brown rice is also good on the side.

1 eggplant
1 red bell pepper
1 yellow bell pepper
1 head broccoli
1 big carrot
1 can unsweetened coconut milk
2 teaspoons hot red Thai curry paste, or more to taste (also comes in a green curry version)
1-inch piece of ginger, minced
3 garlic cloves, minced
2 tablespoons Thai basil, chopped
2 tablespoons cilantro, chopped
Basmati rice for serving

Chop the eggplant, peppers, broccoli, and carrot into bite-sized pieces.

In a wok over medium-high heat, add the coconut milk, and then thoroughly incorporate the curry paste. When the coconut milk starts to simmer, add the vegetables.

Add the ginger, garlic, Thai basil, and cilantro, and cook everything until the vegetables are cooked.

Sweet Orange and Paprika Chicken

Servings: 8 to 12   **Cheats/Serving: 1.5**

½ cup freshly squeezed orange juice
½ teaspoon sea salt
¼ onion, minced
3 garlic cloves, minced
⅛ teaspoon paprika
⅛ teaspoon pepper
4 to 6 boneless, skinless free-range chicken breasts

Mix all the ingredients except the chicken in a resealable food storage bag. Add the chicken and mix to coat the chicken completely. Place the bag in the refrigerator overnight, turning occasionally.

Remove the chicken from the bag, discarding the remaining marinade. Grill over medium heat until tender, about 10 minutes.

SAUCES

Orange Ginger Sauce for Stir-Fry or Fish/Chicken

Servings: 2   **Cheats/Serving: 1**

This is a great sauce for stir-fry. Either add it to your stir-fry at the end of cooking or gently heat it in a saucepan until it turns translucent, about 5 minutes.

2 organic oranges
1 tablespoon vinegar
1 garlic clove (optional)
1-inch piece of ginger (optional)
2 tablespoons frozen orange juice concentrate
2 tablespoons tamari
1 teaspoon sea salt

Remove the zest from one orange.

In a bowl, add the juice of both oranges and the vinegar. Mince the garlic and ginger, if desired, and add to the bowl.

While whisking, add the orange juice concentrate, tamari, and salt.

Peruvian Green Sauce

Servings: 2   **Cheats/Serving: 1**

Serve this on chicken, fish, or pork. It's also great as a topper on any kind of cooked eggs. I also love it on cooked string beans.

Add between 1 and 3 jalapeños, depending on how spicy you like things.

1 bunch (3 ounces) cilantro, stems and all
1 to 3 jalapeños, seeds removed
1 large garlic clove
½ teaspoon salt
2 tablespoons olive oil
2 tablespoons water
1 tablespoon lemon juice

Add ingredients to a food processor and process until smooth

HIGH-NUTRIENT EATS (WITH A LITTLE CHEAT ON TOP)

Brussels Sprouts with Bacon

Servings: 4   **Cheats/Serving: 1**

1 pound Brussels sprouts
1 tablespoon olive oil
3 bacon slices, cooked

Heat enough water to cover the Brussels sprouts to boiling. Add the sprouts and boil for 10 minutes.

Drain the sprouts. When they're just cool enough to handle, cut each one in half.

Heat a pan over medium heat. Add the olive oil. When the oil is hot, sauté the Brussels sprouts until golden brown. Crumble in the bacon and heat through.

Cauliflower Rice

Servings: 2   **Cheats/Serving: 1**

1 head cauliflower
2 tablespoons coconut oil

Process cauliflower until it is the size of rice (use steel blade on food processor, grater or knife). Heat skillet to medium-high heat. Add oil when hot. Saute cauliflower with any seasonings desired (i.e., sea salt, garlic, ginger, curry, black pepper). Stir frequently for 4 to 5 minutes. Serve hot!

Cauliflower with Sweet Onion and Bacon

Servings: 2   **Cheats/Serving: 1**

This recipe was inspired by Cookfresh. It is a yummy, nutrient-dense, detoxifying powerhouse of a recipe that will fill you up and make you feel great. What I like about this recipe is that it uses just one herb in addition to salt and pepper, making it really easy.

If you're craving warm mashed potatoes with bacon, try mashing cauliflower. It has the same consistency as mashed potatoes!

2 slices bacon (feel free to rock your inner bacon if need be)
3 medium garlic cloves, minced or pressed
1 medium sweet onion, thinly sliced into 2-inch-long strips
1 pound chopped cauliflower (usually a large head, chopped into 2-inch pieces)
3 tablespoons chicken broth
1 teaspoon rosemary, finely chopped
1/2 pound fresh spinach leaves
1 teaspoon fresh lemon juice (about 2 squeezes)
Sea salt and fresh ground pepper to taste
1 teaspoon goat cheese (optional)

In a large skillet, cook the bacon over medium-low heat until crisp. Use tongs to take out the bacon and place on a doubled paper towel. Drain most of bacon grease into a bowl. Leave just a bit to cook the rest of the ingredients.

Add garlic, onion, and cauliflower to the skillet, heat over medium heat, and stir until the cauliflower and onion start to turn a golden brown.

Add 2 tablespoons of chicken broth, the rosemary, and the spinach leaves, and cook until cauliflower and spinach are tender, anywhere from 5 to 10 minutes.

Remove from heat. Stir in the bacon, squeeze in the fresh lemon juice, and add salt and pepper to desired taste. If desired, add 1 teaspoon of goat cheese on top.

Garlicky Mashed "Potatoes"

Servings: 2   **Cheats/Serving: 1**

Use butter infused with garlic and spices for an extra flavor in this recipe.

1 large head cauliflower
5 garlic cloves
2 tablespoons grass-fed butter
Salt and pepper to taste

Bring 1 to 2 inches of water to a boil in a stockpot. If you have a steamer insert, have it ready.

Wash and trim the cauliflower, and place it in the steamer (if you're using one) or add it directly to the stockpot. Cover and cook until the cauliflower is soft, about 10 minutes.

Drain the cauliflower very well using a colander. If you don't, your "potatoes" will be watery.

Add the cauliflower to a food processor or blender, and then add the garlic and butter. Process until the cauliflower is smooth. Add salt and pepper.

Perfect Sweet Potato Fries

Servings: 4   **Cheats/Serving: 1**

4 sweet potatoes
4 tablespoons of olive oil
Kosher salt and black pepper to taste
Red pepper flakes to taste

Preheat oven to 450 degrees F.

Cut sweet potatoes in half, keeping the skins on. Cut each half into large slices about ¾ inch thick, and cut those slices into fries ½ to ¾ inches thick.

Put the fries on a baking sheet, making sure they aren't touching. Drizzle olive oil, salt, pepper, and red pepper flakes and mix with your hands, completely covering the sweet potato fries.

Bake in the oven for 15 minutes; after that period, flip and cook for 10 more minutes. You might need less time if you like them less done, or more time if you like them super crispy.

Roasted Broccoli or Asparagus

Servings: 3   **Cheats/Serving: 1**

2 to 3 pounds vegetables: broccoli, asparagus, cauliflower, carrots,
*   zucchini, onion, mushrooms, green beans, beets, rutabaga,*
*   turnips, peppers, whatever!*
3 tablespoons oil
1 teaspoon salt

Preheat oven to 350 degrees F.

Cut all the vegetables into similar-sized pieces. In a large bowl, add the vegetables and oil, and mix well with your hands. Add the salt and mix again.

Spread the vegetables evenly on a cookie sheet or casserole dish (aim for a single layer) and roast for 10 minutes for wet vegetables and 20 to 30 minutes for dense vegetables.

Simple Sautéed Spinach

Servings: 2   **Cheats/Serving: 0**

If your children don't care for spinach, serve mustard or soy sauce on the side for dipping. This trick works great for green beans, too. If you want to add a little more flavor, cup up a couple of garlic cloves and sauté them in the olive oil before adding the spinach.

If you don't have fresh spinach, there is nothing wrong with frozen. Frozen spinach is also cheaper. Overall, spinach is inexpensive and can be very tasty if made right.

2 teaspoons olive oil
8 ounces of prewashed fresh spinach
Red pepper flakes to taste
Sea salt to taste

In a saucepan over medium-high heat, add the olive oil. When it's hot, add the spinach. If your pan isn't big enough, cook the spinach in batches.

Use a wooden spoon or spatula to stir the spinach for about 3 minutes. Add the red pepper flakes and sea salt, and stir for 1 minute. Serve hot.

Sweet Potatoes

Servings: 4   **Cheats/Serving: 0**

4 tablespoons olive oil
4 sweet potatoes
1 large onion, diced
½ teaspoon sea salt
¼ teaspoon freshly ground black pepper

Preheat oven to 400 degrees F.

Pierce the potatoes a few times with a fork and place them on a baking sheet. Bake for 45 minutes, until they're tender.

Meanwhile, heat the oil in a skillet over medium heat. Once it's hot, sauté the onion for 10 to 15 minutes, until it's caramelized.

Once the potatoes are done, cut a slit on the top and add the caramelized onion, salt, and pepper.

Sweet Potato Bacon Bakes

Servings: 4   **Cheats/Serving: 4**

4 tablespoons olive oil
8 pieces grass-fed or nitrate-free bacon
4 large garlic cloves, minced
½ teaspoon sea salt
½ teaspoon pepper
4 medium sweet potatoes
½ cup slivered raw almonds

Preheat oven to 450 degrees F.

Heat 1 tablespoon of the oil in a skillet over medium heat. Add the bacon and cook for 10 minutes.

Meanwhile, in a mixing bowl, combine the remaining oil, garlic, salt, and pepper.

Cut pieces of tinfoil into 4 pieces large enough to wrap each potato loosely.

Rub each potato with the oil mixture, and then wrap each potato in foil and seal by pinching the ends together.

Bake the potatoes on a baking sheet for 40 minutes.

Garnish with the bacon and almonds.

APPS, DESSERTS & EXTRAS

APPETIZERS

Amazing Tart Lime Mango Salsa

Servings: 6   **Cheats/Serving: 1**

My mother-in-law first served a version of this with tangerine on an unusually warm July day in Maine, and as I watched her slave over the tangerine preparation, I thought, wouldn't it be so much easier with mango? The very next day we substituted the mango and voilà! My favorite salsa was born. The mix of the tart lime and the sweet mango are to die for.

This can be used as a topping to tilapia, salmon, or broiled chicken, and it's fantastic on top of a piping-hot bowl of black beans. It's even a great way to cool down a soup or add a boost of flavor to sweet potatoes or squash. I prefer it at room temperature.

Here's the best secret of all: This salsa helps make bad food taste good! If you're invited to a barbecue or dinner, it's a great dish to bring because if you don't care for the fare, you'll have a wonderful topping to mask the mediocre food.

It's a great recipe to keep in the fridge because you can make a large bowl of it and munch all day. With vitamins C and A, mango, and cleansing little cucumber bites, it's a great nutrient addition to any meal.

---

3 mangoes
1 large cucumber
2 tablespoons red onion, finely chopped
¼ cup fresh cilantro, chopped, a bit reserved for garnish
¼ jalapeño, finely chopped
Juice of 1 lime (or more to taste)

Peel the mangoes and slice into 1-inch cubes. Peel the cucumber and cut lengthwise. Scoop out the seeds with a spoon and discard. Dice cucumber into 1-inch cubes. Place in a large bowl. Add cilantro, jalapeño, and lime juice. Sprinkle a bit of the cilantro on top and add a lime wedge for presentation, if desired.

Beef, Chili Beans, and Salsa Mexican Dip

Servings: 6   **Cheats/Serving: 1**

1 pound grass-fed beef
2 cups salsa
One 16-ounce can chili beans, drained
One 2-ounce can sliced olives
½ cup chopped green onion
½ cup chopped fresh tomato

Preheat oven to 350 degrees F.

In a skillet over medium-high heat, cook the ground beef thoroughly. Stir in the salsa, then reduce the heat and simmer for 20 minutes, or until the liquid is absorbed.

Stir in the beans and cook until they're thoroughly heated.

Place the mixture in a bowl and sprinkle the olives, onion, and tomato on top.

Joanie's Artichoke Tapenade

Servings: 4   **Cheats/Serving: 1**

2 garlic cloves
1 handful raw spinach
¼ teaspoon salt
1 fat slice of sweet onion

1 small serrano pepper (or ¼ teaspoon of dried pequin peppers)
20 grinds black pepper
1 tablespoon olive oil
1 tablespoon tahini
2 ounces olives (optional)
1 14-ounce can artichoke hearts, drained
1 large tomato, chopped
2 tablespoons pine nuts
1 handful cilantro (optional)

Add the garlic, spinach, salt, onion, serrano pepper, black pepper, olive oil, tahini, and olives to a food processor and process until it's smooth. Add the artichoke hearts, tomato, pine nuts, and cilantro, and pulse until slightly chunky. Serve immediately.

PEERtrainer Spicy Ranch Dressing with Baked Chicken Wings

Servings: 2   **Cheats/Serving: 7**

This ranch dressing recipe is great because you don't have to have any fresh ingredients—you can just use dried spices and still have your favorite ranch (but without preservatives). It's best paired with grilled barbecue chicken on top of 1 pound of mixed greens.

Spicy Ranch Dressing
4 tablespoons Hellmann's mayo (it must be Hellmann's!)
3 tablespoons apple cider vinegar
¼ teaspoon dried dill weed or herbes de Provence
⅛ teaspoon dried basil
¼ teaspoon dried garlic
¼ teaspoon granulated onion
¼ teaspoon cayenne pepper
⅛ teaspoon salt
⅛ teaspoon pepper

Chicken Wings
3 tablespoons olive oil
2 garlic cloves, pressed
2 teaspoons chili powder
1 teaspoon garlic powder
Salt and pepper to taste
10 chicken wings

Preheat oven to 375 degrees F.

First make the dressing. In a food processor, process the mayo and apple cider vinegar to incorporate. Add the rest of the ingredients and blend well.

Now for the chicken wings, combine the olive oil, garlic, chili powder, garlic powder, salt, and pepper in a large food storage bag. Seal the bag and shake to combine the ingredients.

Add the chicken wings to the bag, reseal, and shake well to coat. Arrange the chicken wings on a baking sheet.

Cook for 1 hour, until crisp and cooked through (no longer dark pink in the middle).

Perfect Mexican Guacamole

Servings: 6   **Cheats/Serving: 1**

This guacamole is great served with thin slices of cucumber or over baked chicken.

2 ripe avocados
1 tablespoon freshly squeezed lime juice
½ teaspoon sea salt
¼ cup thinly sliced green onion
½ cup cilantro, finely chopped
2 tablespoons light or homemade mayonnaise (optional)
1 Roma tomato, diced

Halve the avocados, scoop the flesh into a bowl, and discard the pit. Add the lime juice.

Mash well with a fork or potato masher, and then add the salt, onion, cilantro, and mayonnaise. Once everything is mixed well, fold in the tomatoes.

Pico de Gallo

Servings: 8   **Cheats/Serving: 0**

This piquant sauce from Mexico means beak of a rooster. Traditionally a dip for tortillas, it's a breeze to prepare. Add it to your avocado, quesadillas, black beans, eggs, grilled fish, tuna fish, or hamburgers, or like some aficionados I know, just eat it right out of the bowl. I dip my toasted papadams into this salsa. You can also substitute two ripe mangoes for the tomatoes.

6 Roma tomatoes, chopped
1 small red onion, chopped
¼ bunch cilantro, chopped (or more to taste)
1 jalapeño or serrano pepper (or more to taste)
Juice of 1 lime
¼ teaspoon lime zest
Sea salt to taste

Place all the ingredients in a bowl and mix well.

Shrimp/Lime Appetizer with Parsley

Servings: 2   **Cheats/Serving: 1**

2 handfuls mixed greens
16 jumbo shrimp, cleaned
Juice of 1 lime
8 tablespoons freshly chopped Italian parsley

Place the greens on an appetizer plate and then arrange the shrimp over them. Squeeze the entire lime over the shrimp platter, and then sprinkle the fresh Italian parsley over the top.

Spring Fresh Cherry-Tomato Appetizer

Servings: 4 **Cheats/Serving: 1**

This is a great addition to any traditional protein, like grilled chicken, or atop a bed of mixed greens.

mushrooms
½ pound cherry tomatoes
6 garlic cloves
8 tablespoons cilantro
½ pound artichoke hearts, quartered and rinsed
4 tablespoons olive oil
Juice of ½ lemon
1 to 2 teaspoons red pepper chili flakes (or more to taste)
Salt and pepper to taste
Goat cheese confetti (optional)

Slice the mushrooms, about 4 to 5 slices each mushroom. Halve the cherry tomatoes. Grind the garlic cloves. Chop the cilantro leaves, tossing the stems.

Put the chopped ingredients in a large mixing bowl with the artichoke hearts and olive oil and mix.

Add the lemon juice, red pepper flakes, salt, and pepper, and mix everything well.

Top with goat cheese confetti, if desired.

Toasted Rosemary Almonds

Servings: 6 **Cheats/Serving: 1.5**

1½ cups slivered or sliced almonds
½ teaspoon rosemary
⅛ teaspoon sea salt

Place a large skillet over medium heat. Add the almonds to the skillet and heat until they turn a light golden color and you can start to smell the almond oils, 7 to 10 minutes. Gently stir to allow for even toasting.

Remove from the pan and place in bowl, stirring in rosemary and sea salt.

DESSERTS

Cinna-Raisin Cookies

Servings: 6   **Cheats/Serving: 1**

These cookies make a great after-school treat!

1/2 cup almond flour or almond meal
3 tablespoons walnuts, ground
1 tablespoon ground cinnamon
1/8 teaspoon allspice
1/8 teaspoon nutmeg
1 tablespoon pure raw unfiltered honey
2 tablespoons currants
1/3 cup raisins
1 omega 3–enriched egg

Preheat oven to 350 degrees F.

In a large bowl, mix together the flour, walnuts, cinnamon, allspice, and nutmeg. Add the honey, currants, raisins, and egg, and mix well.

Form small balls and place them on a cookie sheet or baking stone.

Bake for 16 minutes.

Cinnamon Candied Walnuts

Servings: 4   **Cheats/Serving: 2.5**

1½ cups raw walnut halves
⅛ cup organic raw sugar or regular sugar
⅛ teaspoon coarse salt
2 teaspoons of cinnamon

Preheat oven to 350 degrees F.

Lay walnuts out on a baking sheet in a single layer. Bake for 5 minutes. They could need 1 to 2 more minutes; just be careful not to burn the nuts. Make sure you stay in the kitchen to keep your eye on them! After they are toasted, remove them from the oven and let cool.

Pour sugar into a medium saucepan. Cook sugar on medium heat, stirring with a wooden spoon as soon as the sugar begins to melt. Keep stirring until all the sugar has melted and the color is a medium amber to medium caramel color. Immediately add the walnuts to the pan, quickly stirring and coating each piece.

As soon as the walnuts are coated with the sugar, spread them out on a rimmed baking sheet, lined with parchment paper. Use tongs or forks to separate the walnuts from each other, working very quickly. Sprinkle the nuts with the salt and cinnamon.

Easiest Apple Cinnamon Dessert

Servings: 1   **Cheats/Serving: 1**

1 apple, chopped
1 teaspoon raw sugar
1 teaspoon cinnamon

In a small, microwave-safe bowl, mix the apple, sugar, and cinnamon. Microwave for 1 minute on high.

Fantastic Banana Bread

Servings: 12   **Cheats/Serving: 3**

Banana bread on a diet? Yes! This recipe is my mom's. When I realized it had three Cheats a slice, I wanted to see if I could cheatify it. Every recipe I found online either had tons of sugar and fat (one recipe I found had raisins, orange juice, and nuts!) or was so chock-full of chemicals (another recipe had a ½ cup of Equal sugar substitute!) that I couldn't recommend anything else.

If you love banana bread, this recipe is great. It has all natural ingredients and is well worth "spending" five Cheats on!

2 cups all-purpose flour
1 teaspoon baking soda
¼ teaspoon salt
½ cup butter
¾ cup dark brown sugar
2 eggs, beaten
2⅓ cups mashed ripe bananas
1 cup walnuts and pecans (or walnuts and chocolate chips)

Preheat oven to 350 degrees F.

Lightly grease a 9-by-5-inch loaf pan.

In a large bowl, combine flour, baking soda, and salt. In separate bowl, cream together the butter and dark brown sugar. Stir in the eggs and mashed bananas until well blended.

Stir the banana mixture into the flour mixture just enough to moisten everything. Add the nuts and just incorporate them. Pour the batter into the prepared loaf pan.

Bake 60 to 65 minutes, until a toothpick inserted into the center of the loaf comes out clean. Let the loaf cool in the pan for 10 minutes, and then let it finish cooling on a wire rack.

Gajar Halwa

Servings: 8   **Cheats/Serving: 1**

This is a low-fat version of a divine dessert fit for an emperor. Traditionally, it's oozing in ghee and exceedingly sweet. In India, it's served covered with edible silver leaf.

The halwa can be eaten warm or at room temperature.

2 tablespoons ghee or olive oil (not extra-virgin)
1 tablespoon slivered almonds
1 tablespoon unroasted and unsalted pistachios
4 green cardamom pods
4 cups grated carrots
6 tablespoons skimmed milk powder or low-fat ricotta
½ cup organic brown sugar or jaggery (crumbled) if available
2 tablespoons golden raisins (optional)
Rosewater for sprinkling

Heat the ghee in a heavy-bottomed pan over medium heat. When heated, sauté the almonds and pistachios. Remove the nuts and set aside.

Add the cardamom and lightly sauté for 2 minutes.

Add the grated carrots and sauté for 10 minutes or until the liquid is absorbed, stirring frequently so as not to burn.

Add the milk powder, brown sugar, and raisins, and cook until well blended with the carrots.

Cook the mixture over low heat until the ghee pulls away, about 15 minutes.

Remove to a serving dish. Sprinkle the almonds and pistachios on top, and just before serving, sprinkle with rosewater.

PEERtrainer Pumpkin Pie

Servings: 2   **Cheats/Serving: 1**

This recipe can help satiate your sweet tooth as well as give you and your family a huge dose of vitamin A, a critical nutrient in keeping the immune system strong. This can literally be made in a matter of minutes. While lacking the exact flavor and structure of pumpkin pie, if you love pumpkin, this can be a great thing to whip up at the last minute.

Also? Kids love this. (We have proven this in clinical research.)

One 15-ounce can puréed pumpkin
½ tablespoon coconut oil or butter
3 tablespoons sugar or 1 tablespoon molasses (optional)
1 teaspoon cinnamon
⅛ teaspoon powdered ginger (optional)
⅛ teaspoon nutmeg (optional)
Pinch of salt

Put the puréed pumpkin in a microwave-safe bowl. Add the coconut oil and mix. Add the sugar or molasses, cinnamon, ginger, nutmeg, and salt.

Microwave for 3 minutes. Remove, stir, and cool. Add or adjust the flavors as you like.

Raspberry Parfait

Servings: 1   **Cheats/Serving: 2**

1 cup low-fat Greek yogurt
1 cup raspberries
1 tablespoon organic honey
2 teaspoons slivered almonds

Put yogurt in a small bowl, and then top with the other ingredients.

Rj Pops

Servings: 4   **Cheats/Serving: 1**

This recipe calls for Zipzicle bags, which can be purchased at www
.zipzicles.com. If you don't have Zipzicle bags, you can freeze this
recipe in any freezer-proof container. These pops are a fun, refreshing
treat on a warm day.

1 cup fresh or frozen raspberries
⅓ cup coconut milk
1 medium banana
1 tablespoon lemon juice
1 tablespoon pure raw unfiltered honey
1 egg white

In a blender, blend the raspberries, coconut milk, banana, lemon
juice, and honey until creamy.

In a mixing bowl, whisk the egg white with a hand mixer until
peaks have formed.

Pour the raspberry mixture into the mixing bowl and gently fold
in the egg whites.

Using a funnel, pour the mixture into Zipzicle bags and freeze.

Spiced Summer Fruit Compote

Servings: 8   **Cheats/Serving: 1**

Look for cardamom and rosewater at Middle Eastern or Indian grocery stores.

Let your slow cooker cook this light, healthy dessert while you spend the day on the beach or reading in your hammock. Alternatively, you can poach the peaches in a nonreactive saucepan for 30 minutes, or until tender.

1 cup white wine or 1 cup apple or pineapple juice
¼ cup honey
¼ lemon, thinly sliced
2 tablespoons julienned ginger
3 cardamom pods
3 cloves
8 ripe but firm peaches, halved and stones removed
2 cups berries of your choice
Sprinkle of rosewater
Fresh mint leaves for garnish

In a saucepan, heat the wine, honey, lemon, ginger, cardamom, and cloves until bubbling. Add the peaches and spoon the syrup over the top.

Cover and cook over low heat for 90 minutes.

Remove the cardamom, cloves, and lemon slices.

Place the peaches in a serving bowl, pour sauce over the top and gently mix in the berries. Sprinkle with rosewater and garnish with mint leaves.

Watermelon Sorbet

Servings: 2   **Cheats/Serving: 1**

Watermelon is an interesting fruit. It is **relatively** low in calories for a fruit, with roughly 40 to 50 calories per one-cup serving.

There are between 75 and 100 calories in the average slice of watermelon.

Watermelons have a fairly good calorie-to-nutrient ratio. They are rich in vitamin A and C (like most fruit) and also contain some B vitamins, which are thought to be good for energy.

Watermelons also score well on Dr. Fuhrman's system, which factors how many nutrients there are per calorie. Watermelons are rich is a substance called lycopene, which has been shown to be a powerful antioxidant.

This sorbet has no added sugar. It's easy and very inexpensive to make.

4 cups watermelon, cut into chunks
Juice of 1 lime (optional)
1 handful raspberries
1 mint sprig for garnish

Freeze the watermelon overnight.

Place frozen watermelon in a blender and purée until smooth. If you like your sorbet sour, add the lime juice.

Serve topped with raspberries and garnished with mint.

DRINKS

Muscle Recovery Margaritas

Servings: 8   **Cheats/Serving: 2**

This recipe makes enough for a small party. I suggest making the recipe in two stages as the party progresses.

1 bottle Suerte Blanco Tequila
Two 16-ounce bags frozen blueberries
Small amount of fresh ginger (careful—a little goes a long way!)
4 packets Tazo Mint Tea or 2 cups fresh mint
6 to 8 limes
Ice

In a blender, mix ½ bottle of tequila with a bag of frozen blueberries. Add 1 square inch of ginger, the contents of the tea packets or the fresh mint, and the juice of 3 to 4 limes.

Blend until you reach the desired consistency. Add ice to dilute the recipe as needed.

Repeat these steps upon making the second batch.

Nearly Cheat-Free Hot Chocolate

Servings: 1   **Cheats/Serving: 0.5**

1 cup unsweetened coconut milk
1 tablespoon cocoa

Combine ingredients in a small saucepan. Heat on low heat until warm.

PEERtrainer Virgin Piña Colada

Servings: 1   **Cheats/Serving: 1**

1 cup unsweetened coconut milk
½ cup frozen pineapple

Add all the ingredients to a blender and blend until smooth.

Warm Chocolove Hot Chocolate

Servings: 1   **Cheats/Serving: 1**

If you need warm emotional goodness at night, try this recipe inspired by the Chocolove Almonds & Sea Salt in Dark Chocolate bar.

1 cup almond milk
½ tablespoon almond butter
1 date
1 tablespoon unsweetened cocoa powder
1 teaspoon hemp seeds (optional)

Add all the ingredients to a blender and blend on high until smooth. Place the mixture in saucepan and heat until piping hot. You can also microwave it in a microwave-safe container until hot.

———————————————

CHAPTER 10

The Cheat System Maintenance Plan

How to Keep Off the Weight You've Lost—For Good

One of the most important ways to manifest integrity is to be loyal to those who are not present.

—STEPHEN COVEY

You're probably expecting to hear another "plan" in this chapter, including how many Cheats you get to eat and how much exercise you have to do. We'll definitely talk about that, but first I want to discuss the most important part of the maintenance plan: how you're going to keep the weight off long term. (If you can't wait and just want to read the nuts and bolts, you can turn to page 305 for that.)

You've just spent three weeks changing your life. You've been making positive changes for yourself, and maybe even for your family too, and the people around you have noticed. Your friends, who questioned why you were ordering a huge and delicious salad instead of the risotto at dinner, start to ask you what you've done to look so great. The coworker who swears by her tough-as-nails ninety-minute spin class but who still has a belly demands to know what exercise class you took to get rid of yours.

Or maybe you're just on your way there. Maybe you've lost some weight and aren't at your goal weight yet, but you are enjoying how you feel on Cheat System. Or maybe you slipped up a little too often and know that you could do better. Wherever you are, if you've done three weeks on Cheat System, you have succeeded in your goal to make this diet different.

Now is the time for you to figure out how you're going to Cheat and Eat for longer than just three weeks. Even though all the people around you say that they want to know what you've done to look so great, in reality those people will probably end up being the same people who question your good choices going forward. Sometimes your friends, family, and coworkers—really, anyone in your life—will question your choices because it brings up their own issues, which they haven't dealt with. You have to consistently remember what we discussed in Chapter 3: **What other people think about me is none of my business.** But sometimes it's hard. Sometimes slights can really get to us. In those situations, how do you deal?

HOW CAN YOU BE POSITIVE IN A WORLD THAT NATURALLY LEANS NEGATIVE?

I overheard a conversation when I was in Aspen, Colorado, over the summer. Two women were clearly seeing each other for the first time in months. The minute they said "Hi," one complimented the other. "Wow, you look great!"

And the other woman responded, "Are you kidding? Why do I even pay my trainer? Look at the inside of my thighs!"

The other woman replied, "Your thighs? Look at my jiggly arm fat!"

That conversation is typical. I bet you've said something similar. We all do, because as a society, but especially as women, we tend to bond over what's *wrong* with us—what's wrong with our job, what's wrong with our body, our face, our hair—instead of what's actually going *right* and what's amazingly awesome about us. This negativity usually extends past ourselves to other people—it's delicious to exchange gossip, because we get useful information about others in our social circle that way—and getting that view into other people's lives and troubles makes us feel better about our own life.

Most people feel uncomfortable saying positive things about their lives because society has put a total clampdown on talking about success. Talking about your own development and your efforts to better yourself is definitely not considered "cool." It's thought of as bragging by most people. You're never supposed to talk about what you're excited about, whether it's a job or the guy you're dating or your kids excelling in a class or a sport. We're stuck in a place where it's unacceptable to want to improve your life.

I love reading self-help books. When I was in my twenties, I had a stack of self-help books on my nightstand. But when a friend saw my books, she told me to hide them because no guy would ever date me if he saw how many books there were. I ended up hiding *Awaken the Giant Within* by Anthony Robbins, thinking a guy wouldn't be interested in me if I was interested in self-improvement. Today I know that's ridiculous—but I bet you that someone somewhere is hiding her self-help books at this very moment!

For this maintenance plan, I want you to find friends who really are supportive, who are comfortable with you being great. I have made this a must-have in my life, and it's improved my daily life and health dramatically. Whenever I express anxiety or frustration, my friends will remind me of what I want—and how all of those negative things tend to fade away when I concentrate on what's going well in my life.

DON'T RIDE THE NEGATIVE SPIRAL WITH YOURSELF OR WITH OTHERS—FOCUS ON WHAT'S *RIGHT*

In order for you to continue on the path you're on—which is a positive, awesome, life-changing path—you need to make sure you get love and support from people who aren't riding the negative spiral downward.

Just as you have moved away from the Cheats and toward the Eats on your plate, you can begin to tip the scales from the negative to the positive for yourself, your social circle, and even your family. You can start to shift what you bond over with each of your friends and family members, even with your spouse.

This can be tough to do, because our brains are hardwired to focus on what's going wrong (remember, our brains see it as a problem to solve). It's important to remind yourself of what's *right*, what's *working*, what's *good* in your life. That helps you see a hurdle as what it is—an obstacle to get over instead of a giant stop sign. You can start by trying to bond over the smallest positive things, which can be really powerful. Start with one person. Learn how to avoid self-deprecation (and enabling it) by offering that one person help, advice, and ideas instead of falling into the muck.

It might be difficult, especially if you have always connected with your best friend or your spouse or your parent around what's bad or not working in your life. But it's definitely worth trying, because once you find that person who will be positive and offer you support and love without bringing you down, it will give you so much joy and help you keep improving yourself.

BUT WHAT IF ALL MY FRIENDS ARE NEGATIVE?

If finding that person in your life is proving to be a challenge, that's okay. After all, we can't do anything to control other people—even if we are trying to help them make a positive change! If all the people in your life seem to have a cloud over their heads, come visit us at PEERtrainer.com. PEERtrainer was created as a place where people with positive goals could get together and use the power of peer pressure for good (instead of encouraging negative behavior, which it usually does).

So many of our members have succeeded because of the help they received from other people on our forums. You can be completely anonymous if you want; this creates a safe space for you to talk about your struggles, your pain, your concerns, your questions, and your triumphs. Because it's anonymous, people tend to tell the truth. When you have a problem and five people you don't know all offer the same solution and encouragement for you to solve that problem, you will know and trust that those people are telling you the truth. And that's immensely powerful.

THIS IS *YOUR* YEAR

Now is the time for you to focus on you—specifically, on how great you are. The advice in this chapter so far may sound woo-woo or hippie-dippie, but it's really not. (If you try it, you'll see how grounded it is.) At PEERtrainer, we've always challenged people to tackle their relationships and the way they interact with the world at the same time they are tackling their weight, because all of these things are tied to self-identity. Once you start to change one of these elements in your life, your identity begins to shift—and all the other pieces have to shift as well in order to make all the pieces of the puzzle fall into place.

THE REST OF THE PUZZLE

You may have noticed that you have more energy during the day, that you sleep better at night, that the bags under your eyes aren't there anymore, that you are in flow more often than not when you exercise, that you have begun to know instinctively exactly how you're going to Cheat and Eat throughout the day, perhaps even throughout your week. Maybe people have mentioned that you're smiling more, that you have become a positive force in their lives.

These are all ways you can tell that the work you are doing on Cheat System is affecting how you feel long after the initial three-week period you've just been through. This plan is not all about your weight—it's about the problems that your weight was a symptom of. And in order to keep off the weight you've lost, you must be conscious of not only what you eat, how you exercise, and what you weigh but also how you're feeling—so you can avoid slipping back to the place you were at when you started reading this book.

The rest of this chapter focuses on the nuts and bolts: how many Cheats you can have per day when you're in maintenance mode, how you should alter the exercise plan, how to figure out whether you're at the weight you should be, what to do if you suddenly see an increase in the number on the scale, and how to be the best advocate for your own health for the rest of your life. But like the rest of Cheat System, these practical pieces don't make the maintenance puzzle complete without the emotional component. So be sure to monitor how you're feeling as closely as you do the number on the scale.

Tipping the Scale

Earlier in the book, we mentioned that the Cheats and Eats should be seen as two sides of a scale. In maintenance mode, we want you to tip the scale even farther—as far as you can—to the Eats side.

Eating even more Eats will build up the level of micronutrients in your body so that it's easier for your body to recover if and when you mess up or choose to "binge" on Cheats. When you really focus on the Eats, three slices of pizza on Wednesday night with your kids won't automatically mean two more pounds on the scale for the rest of the week.

Though you *can* go up to 10 Cheats per day once you're in maintenance mode, I encourage people to really focus on the Eats. Save your Cheats for a special occasion—the night you want to have pizza with your kids or the evening out with your spouse out. By banking your Cheats and then using them all at once, your body will be more likely to enter a state of equilibrium, which makes it physiologically easier to maintain your weight loss.

Exercise: Build on Your Base

Now that you understand the concept of building your base, you can begin to go faster in your workouts and push yourself more. Just remember what Dr. Phil Maffetone says: Don't get hung up on time. If you've planned to work out for an hour one day, but fifteen minutes in you're starting to stress out about the laundry or your to-do list, and you begin dreading the amount of time you're spending in the workout, stop right there. Personally, I can't even think of doing an hourlong yoga class because twenty minutes in, I always end up worrying about all the things I've got to do that day. But if I just do twenty minutes, it's bliss. Treat your workouts the same.

Also, the more you can change *how* you move—by incorporating different classes, exercises, sports, and activities—the more you will build your complementary muscles, and the better you will look and feel. Try a new sport—if you haven't already done so, try something you liked when you were younger or just something entirely new to you.

My mother went hang-gliding for the first time, and said that it was the thrill of her life and gave her more confidence in her physical abilities. I recently bought the videogame *Just Dance* so I could enjoy movement I love with my daughter.

As Pete Egoscue says, remember how a child moves. They crawl under tables, dig in the dirt, jump up and down, spin in circles, dance like no one's watching. You can also come to PEERtrainer to try more Egoscue exercise menus.

The important thing is that you keep doing what works for you. The Cheat System exercise plan actually doesn't change all that much in terms of *what* you should do (or for how long, because less is more when it comes to exercise), but really *how* you're doing it. Now that you have a base of exercise you're comfortable with—and that doesn't stress your body out—and you have begun to restore your complementary muscles, your workouts should simply build upon that foundation.

Your "Perfect" Weight

This is not a myth. **Everyone has a perfect weight.** You can tell you're at the perfect weight when you have energy, feel good about yourself, and can try on a dress or a pair of jeans without worrying about how they'll fit. You look great in clothes, but your face doesn't look drawn (which can mean you're below your perfect weight).

You know you've reached equilibrium in mind and body when your weight is like a rubber band—it might go up a pound or two after a night out or a vacation, but it's not long before you're back at the right number.

There comes a time where you instinctively know what to eat in any situation, whether it's an office party, having dinner at your in-laws, or being in a hurry and eating Subway for lunch. It's like driving a car: When you first got behind the wheel, you checked your rear-view mirror and your side mirrors and double-checked that everything was right before turning the car on. Now, years later, all those things are automatic and easy for you without much thought. The Cheat System will be the same way.

"HOW OFTEN SHOULD I WEIGH MYSELF?"

This is *very* important, since it helps monitor your progress, or confirm that you're a pound or two away from (remember the rubber band) or are at your perfect weight. At PEERtrainer, some of our members need to weigh themselves every day, while others just do it once a week. (Personally, I do it once a day.)

THE SECRET OF PEOPLE WHO KEEP IT OFF

According to Tony Robbins, people who are successful at weight loss have a number in their head where they want to be. When the number they see on the scale goes up by more than two or three pounds, it sets off an alarm in their head: *Danger! You are off track! Danger! Get back on track!* This is the number one habit of people who have been successful long term at maintaining their weight loss.

I hear what you're thinking: "Jackie, you're so focused on the scale. Shouldn't we be focused on health, because after all, I'm building muscle, and muscle weighs more than fat." And you definitely have a point. I have a neighbor who showed me a picture. She's five feet nine inches and 140 pounds in both photos, but one was taken before she started building muscle and one was taken after. She saw the exact same number on the scale, but she looks drastically different in those photos. Her clothes fit differently, and her body looks transformed.

But here's the truth: whether you're "building muscle" or not, it's important to be comfortable with *your number*. Hitting that number has to make you feel confident in yourself and great overall. When you're not comfortable with your number—when you make it too low or even sometimes too high—you subtly sabotage yourself because you don't really think you can hit it or that it will make you feel awesome. It can be easier to start with a range, or a number you want to be *below.* For some women, it's under 150. For some others, it's under 130. For a lot of guys, it's being under 200 pounds. Whatever it is, try to find your true number or range and stick to it. Keep your weight loss alarm bell set to ready, so that any time you see a number that's two digits higher, it goes off.

What I see a lot at PEERtrainer is that when people have succeeded for a while at losing weight, they forget how hard they've worked to get there. So they slack off or eat more Cheats than normal. Next thing they know, the number they are seeing is 3, 4, 5, maybe even 10 pounds over their number—and those people start to hide. They turn down invitations, they start to miss out on the very things that make us all feel great—connection and fun with our friends.

But that won't happen to you if you keep focusing on the Eats and keep that alarm bell on ready. And don't press the Snooze button. Make it really loud, and when it goes off, get up.

CHAPTER 11

The Cheat System Advanced

How to Get Back on Track or Lose Even More

"Finished last" is always better than "Did not finish," which always trumps "Did not start."

You may have come to this chapter because you're frustrated that you haven't lost more weight or enough weight fast enough. Or maybe you're just curious about what "advanced" really means. Or maybe you're ready to challenge yourself more. Either way, this chapter is for you.

You might be thinking something like "I eat an entire container of spinach at breakfast, a whole head of kale at lunch, and a giant salad for dinner, so I'm definitely going to see the scale drop by two pounds tomorrow." But when you don't, you get frustrated because once again you're doing everything "right" but not losing the weight you expect.

But weight loss doesn't work that way. Weight loss has so many factors, so many reasons for why and how it happens that simple if-then statements rarely come true. (And if it does happen, it's largely coincidental.)

You didn't gain weight in the same exact fashion of two pounds every week for several weeks. And you won't lose weight in that same regimented way, either. Some weeks you'll be down three pounds, some weeks you'll stay the same, and some you'll even gain a pound. *Ugh.* I remember that well.

I want you to try to concentrate on the forest, not the trees. Think about how you feel from day to day. Do you have more energy? Do you feel more optimistic and hopeful? Are you improving your diet, eating fewer Cheats, not snacking or hungry at night? Look at the big picture: Are you doing better? Are you happier? Are you more motivated to change? That means you're moving in the right direction.

YOUR DIET

If the scale is not budging and your belly is not getting smaller, or you're down to the hardest five or ten pounds, the advanced program could be the answer.

First, I want you to take a hard look at how many vegetables you're eating. We've all been so schooled in portion control that sometimes we don't even realize we're doing it, especially with the Eats. It's a habit that dies really, really hard. If you're not eating 80 percent from the Eats side, if you're not eating the equivalent of a family-sized salad bowl or a large mixing bowl full of greens at each of the meals you're eating every day, you're not eating enough of the Eats. Doing that will make a huge difference in your weight loss. You should have your own package of spinach to eat at a meal, your own gigantic salad bowl, your own big plate of greens. Period.

Second, be mindful of how much alcohol, sugar, and caffeine you have in your diet (or even what you used to have). Withdrawal can cause symptoms that mimic hunger, causing you to overeat when actually what your body wants desperately is sleep. If you can, try to replace black teas and coffee with herbal tea or hot water with lemon or herbs like turmeric so you can see if caffeine is part of what's affecting your weight loss.

What's Different About the Advanced?

This chapter takes the Cheat System to a different level. If you're trying to shed weight quicker, this will help. If you're stuck and want to push your body forward, it will also help.

However, because this is advanced, the diet can be stricter. It asks you to eliminate some foods that might be holding you back from losing your hardest pounds.

The actual Advanced Cheat System program is an adapted version of our PEERtrainer Cleanse. We run cleanses at PEERtrainer throughout the year, and I personally do a cleanse four times a year. A cleanse, in our definition, is a tool that "resets" your body. It's not about colonics or drinking only lemon juice with maple syrup and red pepper flakes. A true cleanse is about you eating the most micronutrient-rich food and eliminating any foods that you could potentially be having a physiological reaction to. Our cleanse contains the foods you would eat on a dream day of the normal Cheat System, minus any Cheats.

The Advanced Cheat System plan is ideal for energy, for weight loss, and for truly "cleansing" the body. This version of the diet is similar to spring-cleaning your home. In addition to cleaning the kitchen, making the beds, putting your kids' toys away, and getting organized, you also wash the walls, clean the baseboards, organize the closets, and clean out the cupboards. When you do spring-cleaning, your house is refreshed, inside and out.

Cleanses are a great way to jump-start the Cheat System lifestyle, and are the ideal solution if you find that you're stuck at a plateau with only five or ten pounds to go. However, it's worth noting that cleanses ideally should only be done in moderation.

THE PEERtrainer 14-DAY FRESH START CLEANSE

This advanced cleanse lasts for two weeks, with the option to continue longer if you'd like to evaluate your food sensitivities. It was created by JJ Virgin, and at PEERtrainer we've seen *tons* of success with it.

The Four Foods That Could Be Affecting Your Body and Your Weight Loss

First, this is an elimination cleanse, which means that you cannot eat the following four foods at any point during the cleanse. We remove these foods from your diet because these four foods are the "usual suspects" when it comes to food intolerances and weight-loss resistance.

- ✦ Gluten (found in wheat, rye, and barley)
- ✦ Dairy and eggs
- ✦ Corn and soy
- ✦ GMOs foods (including peanuts)

1. Gluten

Wheat contains a problematic protein: gluten (and specifically, the gliadin part of gluten), which can cause digestive and thyroid problems. For people diagnosed with celiac disease, the symptoms can be severe; many more people have nonceliac sensitivity to gluten, which causes a wide range of symptoms from bloating to runny noses.

You can find out if you are sensitive to gluten by completely eliminating it from your diet. Gluten has been linked to thyroid and autoimmune issues as well, particularly in people who are sensitive. It's also worth noting that wheat doesn't have nearly the nutrition of any Eat on the Cheat Sheet, so eating it could be holding you back from losing more weight.

If you eliminate gluten, do not substitute "gluten-free" foods. Most of these are made with the other culprits, such as corn or soy. If you want to go gluten-free (I have very low levels of wheat/gluten in my diet), try quinoa or rice as an alternative to gluten *and* "gluten-free" food).

2. Dairy and Eggs

Like soy and corn, dairy used to be okay for us to eat—before food companies began to alter how it was made and processed.

Today, in addition to the fact that most people are lactose-intolerant, the type of cow most farmers and agricultural companies use to produce milk and cheese—the Holstein—produces a type of casein protein that causes digestive problems. Though you can get cow's milk that doesn't have this protein, it's rare to find in the United States. So if you've been including milk, cheese, or other dairy as Cheats, try eliminating them altogether. If you have skin issues, it would be a good test to eliminate dairy.

3. Corn and Soy

Corn and soy don't cause problems when eaten as condiments, but over the past few decades both have become so processed that these formerly healthy foods tend to pack on the pounds.

Soy is touted as a "complete protein." This may be true, but in order to achieve high levels of protein in soy products, the soy protein is isolated. This doesn't cause a problem if you eat small amounts, but if you're relying on soy products to make up the majority of the protein in your diet—as many vegans and vegetarians do—it can cause harm. Many people mistakenly eat soy because they reference studies long ago of women in Japan who have low incidences of breast cancer. First, they are eating a different kind of soy: fermented soy. Second, the Japanese actually don't eat large amounts of soy. They eat it as a condiment. So if you love soy, just look at it as a condiment and have it only a couple times a week.

Corn has a similar story. It's important to keep in mind that corn is *not* a vegetable—it's a grain! Corn simply does not have the same power to improve health that vegetables do. Corn also ends up being processed and put into foods that never had corn in their natural state, which can cause problems for people in terms of losing weight. Be sure to avoid *anything* with corn syrup (especially high-fructose corn syrup) while on the Advanced Cheat System.

Soy and corn should be viewed as condiments or Cheat Confetti, not as staples of your diet. While having some tempeh at an Asian restaurant won't cause you any harm, replacing all your protein with soy will harm more than help. The same applies to corn: while an occasional ear or corn tortilla won't pack on the pounds, eating foods that are processed from corn definitely will. When in doubt, keep corn and soy out!

4. GMOs

GMOs—genetically modified organisms—are modified expressly to survive being sprayed with herbicides, which affect our health when we eat them. And unfortunately, the more vegetables we ingest, the more toxic herbicides enter our body and affect its processes.

Thankfully, there's an easy way to avoid GMOs—buy 100 percent certified organic food. Certified organic food by law cannot contain GMO ingredients.

Though organic is usually better than conventional produce, there are so many factors to how food is grown—from the soil it's in to the growing conditions of a given season—that it's hard to tell what's really better. Additionally, many farmers and products are actually producing organic grade produce and goods but simply don't have the finances to become "certified organic." Don't worry if you can only afford conventional or if the organic section at your grocery store has been picked over. Eating a conventionally grown pepper is better than eating mac and cheese any day.

Another way to avoid GMOs in all of your foods is to buy local and in season. It's better for your health and your weight loss to eat produce that's raised locally and harvested at the time nature intended.

Detoxifying Protein Shakes

Second, during the cleanse you will drink two protein shakes every day, with a meal, for lunch or dinner. You should space out how often you eat or drink protein shakes by about four to six hours so your body can properly detoxify.

Your protein shakes should be made from a pea and rice protein combination, or some other *complete* vegan protein powder such as brown rice protein. Do not use protein powder made from whey, egg, casein, or soy, because these are eliminated foods. The protein shake should have at least 20 grams of high-quality protein. Mixing in a fiber supplement is highly recommended as well (at least 5 grams of soluble fiber per shake is best).

A Cleansing Meal

Third, for lunch or dinner you will eat a meal. This meal is composed of four different things:

+ 4 to 6 ounces of clean, lean protein (6 to 8 ounces for larger/ more athletic women, 8 to 10 ounces for men)
+ 1 to 2 servings of a healthy fat (e.g., 1 tablespoon olive oil, ¼ an avocado, 10 nuts, or 4 ounces fish per serving)
+ 2+ servings of nonstarchy vegetables (serving size is ½ cup cooked or 1 cup raw)
+ 1 serving of high-fiber starchy carbs (½ cup beans or rice, ½ a sweet potato, 1 piece of fruit). *Note: Starchy carbs are only allowed for the first week!*

If you are hungry and need to have a snack, it should be something high in protein, healthy fat, and nonstarchy vegetables. Nuts and cut vegetables are be great, as is nut butter on celery sticks. A small serving of turkey and vegetables is also be fine.

Because this cleanse is meant to eliminate toxins, it's recommended that you slowly wean yourself off substances that need to be detoxified by the body, including caffeine and alcohol. That doesn't mean you have to go cold turkey, though! Just slowly lessen your consumption. So, for example, if you normally drink two cups of coffee a day, you should start by switching to drinking two cups of half-caffeinated coffee, then drop down to one cup. If you have two glasses of wine a night, go down to one glass.

If you find that you "need" caffeine to wake up, green tea is preferred. Switching from coffee or black tea to green tea is great because it's the best of both worlds: it allows your body to detoxify and allows you to get your fix. But switching isn't required.

Alcohol also isn't totally prohibited, though some alcoholic beverages are worse than others. Keep in mind that most beers contain gluten, so beer is definitely not allowed unless it is certified gluten-free. Red wine is okay, but it's important to avoid alcohols that are by nature sweet. It's also better to buy higher-quality alcohol during the cleanse, because the processing is better. Opt for less of the better stuff.

THE CLEANSE, WEEK BY WEEK

Week One

During the first week, you should drink two protein shakes a day and eat one meal that includes a serving of starchy carbs. If you are starving and need a snack it's okay to have one, but try to avoid it. The first week is typically the hardest: you might have headaches and other withdrawal symptoms from foods like sugar. These symptoms usually dissipate after a few days, but if they do not, it is always recommended to see a doctor to ensure that there is nothing more serious happening!

Week Two

The second week is nearly the exact same as the first week, with one exception: your one regular meal each day is no longer allowed to have any starchy carbs! Instead, increase the amount of nonstarchy vegetables you eat.

Week Three

Your cleanse is officially done after Week Two, but if you think you might have food sensitivities, you can begin to test that in Week Three. One of the advantages of eliminating foods is that you can reintroduce them one at a time to see whether they are problematic for you or not. The most important thing here is to do them only *one at a time*, so you can be absolutely sure which foods are causing symptoms!

Testing Your Food Sensitivities

When you want to test a new food, introduce it into your diet for three to four days. Keep track of your symptoms! If you develop new symptoms (such as a runny nose) when you introduce the food, and this symptom goes away when you eliminate it again, then you are probably sensitive to that food. If you experience no symptoms, then that food is probably fine.

Take the time to go through all six foods on the bulleted list at the beginning of the cleanse section. Test a food for four days, and then eliminate it for three before trying a different food.

If you are sensitive to a food, keep it out of your diet for at least six months before rechallenging it. Many food sensitivities can resolve over time, so rechallenging foods from time to time can allow you to check whether you have reversed your sensitivity. If you fail again after six months, you should eliminate the food again for a year before rechecking!

THREE FOODS THAT COULD BE HOLDING YOU BACK

In addition to the foods restricted on the Advanced Cheat System Cleanse, there are three other foods that sometimes restrict weight loss: beans and pseudo-grains like quinoa, smoked foods, and healthy fats.

BEANS AND PSEUDO-GRAINS

If you're having trouble losing weight, it could be the beans or the seeds. Though technically these foods are free, many people don't digest these foods well, so very large portions can hold you back from losing weight. Try eliminating beans from your diet and see if it helps. If it does, consider beans and seeds as Cheats.

SMOKED FOODS

Smoked foods—from barbecue to smoked salmon—can be high in compounds called polycyclic aromatic hydrocarbons, or PAHs. These compounds are toxic and cause a number of health problems. In general, smoked fish is less healthy for you than unsmoked fish—so if you're struggling with your weight, try eliminating all smoked foods from your diet.

HEALTHY FATS

If you're struggling with your weight, it can be helpful to avoid eating too many high-fat foods like nuts, seeds, and coconut milk. Though all of these foods contain healthy fats that are good for you, it's still fat—which your body may be storing, instead of burning—especially if you're not following the Cheat System Exercise Plan from Chapter 3.

However, it's important to still include a healthy fat in each meal so that you will feel satiated and be able to wait for your next meal to eat again.

EXERCISE

Are You Really at Your Base?

If you're struggling with your weight, you may still be working out over your base. Since this is the advanced program, I'd urge you to get a heart rate monitor. This is a great way to tell if you're burning fat or if you're above your base and just burning sugar (which causes you to have excess cortisol and store more fat than you should).

Here's how to tell what your heart rate should be when you're working out at your base level. I learned this formula from both Stu Mittleman and Phil Maffetone: Subtract your age from 180. Go down by 10. That range is your base.

For example: If you're forty years old, you would subtract 40 from 180, which is 140. Go down by 10. Your fat-burning state is between 130 and 140. It's okay to increase the intensity of your workout at the end, or for 15 percent of the overall workout—so your heart rate during that period will be higher, probably over 140.

It can also be helpful to retake the quiz in Chapter 3. If you answered yes to four or more of those questions, the likelihood that you're working out above your base level is very high and your body is in a high cortisol state, which could be holding you back from losing more weight. The heart rate monitor is the single best tool to actually measure if this is what you're doing.

EXERCISE BELLY

If you're working out and properly Cheating and Eating, but you still haven't seen a noticeable difference in your belly, you are probably overtraining. I want you to work out one less day a week. If you are working out five days, do four. You have to take overtraining seriously and reset the way you're exercising if you want to get rid of the extra weight you're carrying in your belly.

Build Your Complementary Muscles More

I'd like you to increase the amount of childlike movement in your exercises so that you build your complementary muscles in different ways than the Egoscue stretches do.

A great exercise to try is hiking. It's a great way to build complementary muscles and get a fat-burning workout. Most of the time you can't hike fast and there are always obstacles to climb around, which will engage muscles you're not used to using. There's a reason so many people in Boulder, Colorado, are so fit. Most of the sports inherent to the area require you to move in all different ways: step on this rock, avoid getting your shoe wet in the creek.

Whatever you do, try to mix it up: When you keep doing the same sport as your primary exercise, whether that's basketball or tennis or running, you're going to be using the same muscles over and over again. If you change up what you do, your body will react differently.

Another great "exercise" to try is meditative breathing. Meditation has a terrible reputation for being boring or sort of woo-woo, but it doesn't have to be. Meditation doesn't have to mean crossing your legs or chanting a mantra. Meditation can be listening to music while sitting in a park. Meditation can mean sitting on your bed and staring out your window, just letting your thoughts take over.

Meditation trains you to let go internally. It's a time-out for you. And that's really important. Though we all want to strangle the person who tells us to "relax," we all do need five minutes to ourselves in order to reset our stress and hormone levels. When you're pressed for time, five minutes of meditation will be better exercise for weight loss than doing twenty minutes on a treadmill that you'd spend worrying about getting your workout in and still getting your to-do list done.

THE PEERTRAINER SUCCESS INDEX

One tool our members love is seeing their number on the PEERtrainer Success Index. It's a quick survey, but it's unlike any weight-loss survey you've taken before, and it measures where you actually are on the road to successful weight loss.

Come find out your number. Go to success.peertrainer.com to get your score. Your score helps you see where you are on the Cheat System scale. Most important, take the quiz again after the three weeks! You'll be surprised at how much your number changes.

The Brain and the Body

An intrepid physician we recently partnered with at PEERtrainer named Dr. Eric Cobb has found that sometimes injury lasts far longer than we think—sometimes years, even decades. That's because injury can block the neural pathways that connect your brain to your joints and muscles. If you picture these pathways as roads, what injury does is create a traffic jam. Even after the injury is healed, the roadblock remains.

After seeing patients come in over and over again with the same pain symptoms, Dr. Cobb set out to find a different way of recovery training that would have a lasting effect. In his opinion, Dr. Cobb didn't go through years of training just to be the aspirin people relied on. So he did some research and some testing and came up with a system called Z-Health. He designed a training system that doesn't focus on our muscles but rather on what's really holding you back: the traffic jam blocking your brain from communicating with the rest of your body.

Z-Health exercises, including the three that are part of the Advanced Cheat System stretches, work on repairing the roads between our muscles and our brain so you can be pain-free and have the ability to do more. The exercises may seem strange or more simple than you're used to, but it's proven to work. Over 70,000 trainers around the world practice Z-Health techniques with their clients.

THE PEERtrainer CHEAT SYSTEM Z-HEALTH EXERCISES

The secret to reaching your physical goals is found in how fluently your brain and your body are communicating with each other. There are three primary systems that contribute to the "brain language" between your brain and your body when it comes to control and coordinating physical activity, including performing athletic activities:

Your eyes (the visual system)
Your inner ear (the vestibular system)
Your joints, muscles, and nerves (the proprioceptive system)

Because these systems are incredibly intricate and interconnected, small problems in any one of them can affect all three—creating huge problems like pain, inflexibility, poor posture, and a lack of coordination. That's why we think fixing these problems is so important, and we fix each by training each system.

1. Train the Eyes (The Visual System)

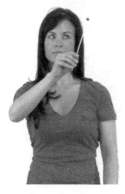 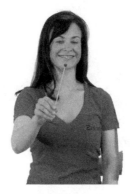

This drill trains and exercises your ability to smoothly track objects in the full range of your visual field. Both visual strength and coordination are required to do this well.

Stand in a comfortable position, feeling balanced and relaxed.

Hold your finger, a pen, or other visual target in front of your nose.

While keeping your head as still as possible, start making a spiral close to your face. Slowly move your finger away from your face out to arm's length, gradually increasing the size of the spiral.

For thirty seconds, move the spiral away from you.

For another thirty seconds, move the spiral toward you.

Repeat in a vertical direction. Start with your pen or your finger near your navel. Slowly spiral up for thirty seconds until your eyes are looking up.

Repeat the spiral in the opposite direction back down to the starting position.

2. Train the Inner Ear (The Vestibular System)

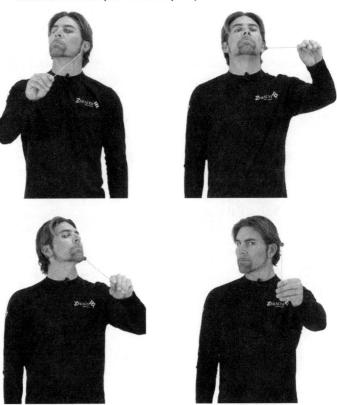

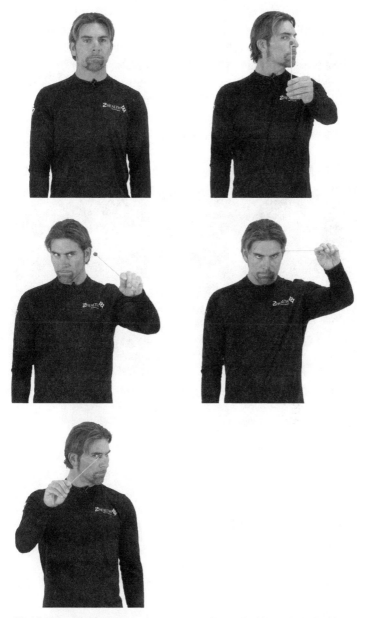

This drill trains the ability to stabilize your eyes on a target when your head is in motion. During this exercise, your visual picture should remain clear throughout the head movements. If it becomes blurry or doubles, restart the exercise and move more slowly.

Stand in a comfortable position feeling balanced and relaxed.

Attempt to *smoothly* move your head in a straight line following one of the directions shown in the figures *while keeping your eyes fixed* on a target in front of you. Then return the head to a neutral position.

Perform three repetitions in each direction. Perform only one direction at a time, which results in eight sets of three repetitions each.

If you notice excessive sway or an inability to keep your eyes on the target while performing the drill, you can also do it sitting down.

3. Train the Joints, Muscles, and Nerves (The Proprioceptive System)

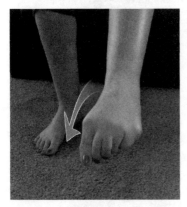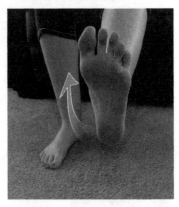

This drill trains the muscles, joints, and nerves of your feet to work together in a movement sequence. Your feet are (in most cases) the first part of the body to meet the ground during athletic activity. Our feet experience a lot of force and absorption, so it is vitally important that we have good active control of our feet in multiple directions.

Sit or stand in a comfortable position, feeling balanced and relaxed.

Lift one foot off the floor.

Attempt to *smoothly* curl your toes, your foot, and point your ankle toward the floor. Then reverse directions and uncurl the toes, extend the foot, and point the ankle toward the sky.

Repeat three to five repetitions of the wave on each foot.

Do not move into sharp pain. If you feel pain, either slow down or decrease your range of motion.

IF YOU'RE STILL NOT SEEING RESULTS

It might be your hormones. When our hormones are at normal and healthy levels, our body functions just how it should. Weight gain and fatigue are much less common. But when our hormones are out of whack—or when they've been that way for a long time—losing weight can be hellish.

As we've taught you throughout the book, cortisol plays a huge role in weight. When cortisol increases when you exercise or are feeling stressed, it tells the body to save all remaining blood glucose (sugar) for the brain. It increases insulin resistance in our muscles, so muscles don't use any of the glucose. And it breaks down the protein in our muscles in order to create new glucose cells in the liver. While these processes are essential for exercise—otherwise we'd pass out from our brain not having enough glucose—these processes can be your weight-loss problem.

Because there's no extra demand for energy other than when we exercise, all cortisol does is cause our blood sugar to rise and our body to store the glucose it just created in our liver—growing our fat stores. And to make things worse, every time we do that, we increase the insulin sensitivity in our fat cells, encouraging our body to store extra calories there. Remember, that process happens when we stress out. So stress is not just uncomfortable but can cause us to store fat.

But cortisol isn't the only hormone that can cause us to gain weight (or not lose any) when it goes out of whack. Our thyroid also secretes hormones that can make it easier or harder to lose weight. Our thyroid is often called the "master switch for our metabolism" because it so directly controls whether our metabolism runs fast, slow, or just right. When our thyroid stops secreting optimal amounts of certain thyroid hormones, our metabolism can slow to a crawl. We end up feeling fatigued and naturally burn fewer calories each day.

Unfortunately, getting our thyroid hormones back to normal isn't simple. If you think this may be you, as much as it might stress you out to take the time to see a doctor, do it anyway. As Dr. Sara Gottfried repeats over and over, "It's easier to fix your problems than it is to live with them." And she's right.

There isn't a single solution that will help improve your thyroid levels, but a couple of remedies to consider include optimizing your vitamin D levels, giving up gluten, and avoiding goitrogenic foods—particularly soy and members of the cabbage family (including broccoli, sadly).

Estrogen could also be a factor in why you're not losing weight. When there's too much estrogen in our body, you can be more prone to accumulating fat on your bum and thighs. There are a few types of estrogen, some good, some bad. The ultimate goal is to lower the bad estrogens and increase the good. If you suspect your hormones might be out of whack at all, it would be wise to give up alcohol. Though alcohol doesn't cause problems for people with overall healthy hormonal levels, it does increase cortisol and "bad" estrogen, especially when consumed regularly over time. If you're struggling to lose that last five to ten pounds, give up the alcohol (as hard as that is!) for at least a month to help your hormones return to healthy levels and to give your body the best shot at shedding all of its extra weight.

SEE A DOCTOR . . .

If you have been doing the Cheat System for three weeks and have not seen your weight decrease by more than two pounds, see a doctor. That is a big indicator that something more substantial might be happening with your hormones.

ONE LAST THING

When you're doing the Advanced Cheat System, I would love you to create a vision board. It might seem completely cheesy, and if you'd ever done one and told people about it, you might have gotten a lot of comments. But most successful CEOs use a whiteboard so they can visually lay out what they intend to do with their business. It works—

and you don't have to show it to anyone. In fact, I don't want you to show it to anyone, because your vision board is personal. Seeing something that personal tends to make others uncomfortable, even if it's a spouse.

Your vision board is all about you. You can cut out pictures, write down words, copy inspirational quotes you like, anything you want—just so long as it represents the direction you want to go in. Putting your thoughts on paper will marry your focus with your goals—and will push you toward success. You're the CEO of your diet and your body and your health—so there's no reason you shouldn't have a vision board like the most successful CEOs in business.

Conclusion: Why You *Can* Lose Weight Now

Twenty years from now you will be more disappointed by the things that you didn't do than by the ones you did do.

—MARK TWAIN

You might be thinking, "Okay, Jackie, but how am I actually going to do this. I understand it's a list. I eat as much as I want from the Eat side and I just count my Cheats. I stop burning myself out and beating myself up when I haven't gotten to the gym. And I can still eat my cheese and lose weight. But I've tried this before. I have every best intention to start on Monday and I get thrown off. Or I'm great all day and I mess up at night. Why is this going to be different? How can I really do it this time? Because I need to. I have to do this. I want to look good. I want to feel good. I want to be back where I know I'm in the zone and I'm getting it done."

I think this happens to almost everyone who reads a diet book. You read the entire thing, thinking the whole time, "This all sounds great, but can I really do it?" You can. You will succeed on the Cheat System. Here's why:

NOTHING IS OFF THE TABLE

If you really love your coffee with Splenda in the morning or having a glass of wine in the evening, you don't have to give that up. You simply just have to count it as a Cheat. Nothing is ever off-limits, period.

The Cheat System is a list—with everything included. We've designed the system so that we do the work for you. You eat your Eats and limit your Cheats, with a few exceptions to the rules. Your focus on Eats will negate the body blows of the Cheats, and this will become so automatic, you won't even think about it. You aren't focused on fiber or fat or nutrients. We've done that for you. You eat your Eats, and you limit your Cheats.

THERE'S NO SUCH THING AS FAILURE

If you sat on the couch all week, you can still succeed on this diet. If you binged on potato chips last night, you can still succeed on this diet. Whatever you feel like you did that was "bad" or "wrong" can be overcome on this diet.

When you accept that you can't fail, no matter what, you will be able to shift your focus from what you are unable to do or are doing "wrong" to what's possible, doable, and going *right*. When you shift your focus, it's far easier to follow through and succeed.

You don't have to beat yourself up anymore because you haven't embraced the latest churn-and-burn craze. You don't have to feel bad that you ate a piece of bread. You will feel good about your small successes, and they will lead to you losing the weight.

THE WEEKLY ONE THING

The weekly one thing is a great solution for people who have no idea where to start. The thought of starting anywhere seems too overwhelming. If you're thinking, "How can I do this? I have three kids, I've done this before, everything I try doesn't work, I'm great all day but then I mess up at night, I am in so much trouble at work, maybe I can start this in three weeks," then this is the solution for you.

When you're in the middle of living your life, figuring out where to start can be really tough. That's why I asked you at the beginning of the book to pick just one thing that's tripping you up. Did you pick that one thing and focus on changing it? If so, what was it? Were you successful? How did that make you feel? Can you pick one more thing that you want to start changing?

Whether you participated in that "one thing" exercise at the beginning or not, now is the time for you to pick something. If you're not sure where to start, simply focus on one thing that's tripping you up and focus on changing that one thing. It can be anything: late night snacking, avoiding donuts at the office, not buying potato chips, whatever. You don't have to fix everything all at once; you start by picking just one thing.

When you put your energy and your focus into changing this one thing, you will change how you feel. And if you turn the one thing into a weekly one thing—changing one thing a week about your diet or lifestyle—you will slowly build momentum and transition into a mode that is hopeful. I don't know how else to describe it—I actually call it "hope mode" with my PEERtrainer members. Being in hope mode is so powerful; it will make every challenge seem conquerable and make you feel undefeatable. And it all starts with just one thing.

You can do this, and you will do this—because this is *your* year.

What do I mean by that? I mean that *this* is the year you're going to make a change. *This is the year you will succeed.* Write "this is the year" on a piece of paper and tape it to your mirror, put it in your phone as an alarm, turn it into a mantra: This is the year. This is the year. This is the year. This is *my* year.

That's the truth. It *is* your year. What you've done in the past—the failures, the successes, everything that could have been—has all built to this coming year, when things will be different. This is the year when things will change. You might be reading this in November or May or August. It doesn't matter, because the next 365 days are all about you. In those next 365 days, your life, your weight, and your happiness will change. Because the Cheat System will give you momentum that you haven't had before, the momentum you need to make this *your* year.

This is not the year to *think* about this being the time for what you're going to do or what you want to do in your life; this is the year to *do* everything you've wanted. This is your year—and I promise you that once you begin to take that on, you will experience flow and fly. You will experience more daily success than you have before, and will build the momentum and push to accomplish all the goals you want to over the next year.

Believing that this is your year helps you live in the mode of hope. It gets you in your zone. When you're in the zone, bang-ups and hang-ups still happen to you, but you quickly remind yourself that this is the year. You get that feeling, that special knowing feeling that things are going to be different this time.

This is the year when you make the change. This is your year to be successful by focusing on the Eats and choosing your Cheats. It's just that simple. Focus on the list and balancing the scale of how many Eats you eat in a day versus Cheats. You can do this and you are going to do this. You don't need to worry about fat, fiber, calories, or anything other than what you've learned. And, most important, remember that when you focus on eating the Eats, the Cheats take care of themselves. **You can do this. And you will! This is the year.**

Appendix:
The Cheat System for Athletes

If you're an athlete working out more than the average person, the Cheat System changes in terms of diet. How you alter the plan is ultimately dependent on your goals, but if you want to lose weight, the plan won't change all that much. (However, if you're interested in improving performance goals, you might need to change the plan further.)

First, if you are an athlete you may need to eat more. If you find that you don't have the energy to do your normal workout routine or regular activities, try increasing the amount of nonstarchy vegetables that you eat. These are Eats, so it really doesn't have that great an effect on the diet or number of Cheats you use each day. If that doesn't work, increase the amount of starchy carbohydrates you eat.

Because athletes work out harder and longer than most people, their workouts tend to deplete more sugar reserves. Eating about half to one cup extra of starchy carbohydrates, like beans, during a meal will provide the replenishment those glycogen stores need. Seeds and nuts are your friend here. Use these nutrient boosters as well.

It can also be helpful to eat more protein at certain times of the day. If you eat breakfast at 8 A.M., have lunch at noon, and then eat dinner at 6 P.M. or later, drinking a protein shake around 3 or 4 P.M. in the afternoon can help ensure that your body is getting enough protein to recover and maintain the improvements in performance that your workouts should create.

However, the afternoon "snack shake" shouldn't become a meal, because that adds too many calories to your daily diet and will counteract any benefit you get from the protein. The snack shake should simply be made of protein; no fat and no carbs are necessary. Consuming just protein at this time in the day will stimulate fat-burning mode, whereas having a full meal in shake form will only tell the body that it should store any excess calories as fat (exactly the opposite of what you want for effective weight loss!).

This is really only relevant to athletes. An increase in protein for the average person, uncoupled with exercise, will not help you lose weight or build muscle. At best, it will be a neutral meal. At worst, the protein will be so unnecessary that all of it will just be oxidized for energy, offsetting the energy that might have been burned from fat. The point is that you need to eat extra protein throughout the day only if you create a deficit—in other words, if you have a well-established base fitness and do hard, long, or intense workouts.

Bibliography

Bell, E. A., and B. J. Rolls. 2001. Energy density of foods affects energy intake across multiple levels of fat content in lean and obese women. *American Journal of Clinical Nutrition* 73(6): 1010–1018.

Ello-Martin, J. A., J. H. Ledikwe, and B. J. Rolls. 2005. The influence of food portion size and energy density on energy intake: Implications for weight management. *American Journal of Clinical Nutrition* 82(1): 236S–241S.

Fuhrman, J., B. Sarter, D. Glaser, and S. Acocella. 2010. Changing perceptions of hunger on a high nutrient density diet. *Nutrition Journal* 9: 51.

Hill, E. E., E. Zack, C. Battaglini, M. Viru, A. Viru, and A. C. Hackney. 2008. Exercise and circulating cortisol levels: The intensity threshold effect. *Journal of Endocrinological Investigation* 31(7): 587–591.

Jeffery, R. W., R. R. Wing, C. Thorson, L. R. Burton, C. Raether, J. Harvey, and M. Mullen. 1993. Strengthening behavioral interventions for weight loss: A randomized trial of food provision and monetary incentives. *Journal of Consulting and Clinical Psychology* 61(6): 1038.

Koziris, L. P., W. J. Kraemer, S. E. Gordon, T. Incledon, and H. G. Knuttgen. 2000. Effect of acute postexercise ethanol intoxication on the neuroendocrine response to resistance exercise. *Journal of Applied Physiology* 88(1):165–172.

Kral, T. V., and B. J. Rolls. 2004. Energy density and portion size: Their independent and combined effects on energy intake. *Physiology and Behavior* 82(1): 131–138.

Ledikwe, J. H., H. M. Blanck, L. K. Khan, M. K. Serdula, J. D. Seymour, B. C. Tohill, and B. J. Rolls. 2006. Dietary energy density is associated with energy intake and weight status in U.S. adults. *American Journal of Clinical Nutrition* 83(6): 1362–1368.

Li, Y., C. Wang, K. Zhu, R. N. Feng, and C. H. Sun 2010. Effects of multivitamin and mineral supplementation on adiposity, energy expenditure and lipid profiles in obese Chinese women. *International Journal of Obesity* 34(6): 1070–1077.

Lichtman, S., et al. 1992. Discrepancy between self-reported and actual caloric intake and exercise in obese subjects. *New England Journal of Medicine* 327(27): 1893–1898.

Madsen, E. L., A. Rissanen, J. M. Bruun, K. Skogstrand, S. Tonstad, D. M. Hougaard, and B. Richelsen. 2008. Weight loss larger than 10% is needed for general improvement of levels of circulating adiponectin and markers of inflammation in obese subjects: A 3-year weight loss study. *European Journal of Endocrinology* 158(2): 179–187.

Moorhead, S. A., R. W. Welch, M. Barbara, E. Livingstone, M. McCourt, A. A. Burns, and A. Dunne. 2006. The effects of the fibre content and physical structure of carrots on satiety and subsequent intakes when eaten as part of a mixed meal. *British Journal of Nutrition* 96(3): 587–595.

Rojas Vega, S., H. K. Strüder, B. Vera Wahrmann, A. Schmidt, W. Bloch, and W. Hollmann. 2006. Acute BDNF and cortisol response to low intensity exercise and following ramp incremental exercise to exhaustion in humans. *Brain Research* 1121(1): 59–65.

Rolls, B. J., E. A. Bell, and M. L. Thorwart. 1999. Water incorporated into a food but not served with a food decreases energy intake in lean women. *American Journal of Clinical Nutrition* 70(4): 448–455.

Rolls, B. J., et al. 1998. Volume of food consumed affects satiety in men. *American Journal of Clinical Nutrition* 67(6): 1170–1177.

Rolls, B. J., L. S. Roe, and J. S. Meengs. 2004. Salad and satiety: Energy density and portion size of a first-course salad affect energy intake at lunch. *Journal of the American Dietetic Association* 104(10): 1570–1576.

Soni, A. C., M. B. Conroy, R. H. Mackey, and L. H. Kuller. 2011. Ghrelin, leptin, adiponectin, and insulin levels and concurrent and future weight change in overweight postmenopausal women. *Menopause* 18(3): 296.

Van Bruggen, M. D., A. C. Hackney, R. G. McMurray, and K. S. Ondrak. 2011. The relationship between serum and salivary cortisol levels in response to different intensities of exercise. *International Journal of Sports Physiology and Performance* 6(3): 396.

Wansink, B., J. E. Painter, and J. North. 2005. Bottomless bowls: Why visual cues of portion size may influence intake. *Obesity Research* 13(1): 93–100.

Wing, R. R., R. W. Jeffery, L. R. Burton, C. Thorson, K. Sperber Nissinoff, and J. E. Baxter. 1996. Food provision vs structured meal plans in the behavioral treatment of obesity. *International Journal of Obesity* 20(1): 56–62.

Yao, M., and S. B. Roberts. 2001. Dietary energy density and weight regulation. *Nutrition Reviews* 59(8): 247–258.

Acknowledgments

There were so many people who helped me create the Cheat System and this book. A special thanks to my husband, Habib Wicks, and my mom, Joan Divine. I could not have done this without you. Also special thanks to Michael Divine, Sukanya Rahman, and Frank Wicks. And Jake and Sarah, who love to play the Cheats/Eats game in the grocery store

I also want to thank friends and colleagues, in no order of importance. I love and appreciate you all: Brian Rigby, Anthony Robbins, J.J. Virgin, Brian Bradley, Dr. Srini Pillay, Pete Egoscue, Dr. John Sarno, Fred Nazem, Marty Seligman, Dr. Sara Gottfried, Dr. Daniel Amen, Leanne Ely, Dr. Eric Cobb, Jonathan Fields, Dr. Steven Masley, Michael Fishman, Michael Lovitch, Phil Maffetone, Marc Stockman, Blake Kassel, Joshua Wayne, Daniel Goleman, Brendan Burchard, Mitchell Stevko, Olga Stevko, Ryan Adams, and Katie Martin. And a gigantic thank you to our editor, Nichole Argyres, our collaborator, Meghan Stevenson, and our agent, Celeste Fine.

Finally, to all of our PEERtrainers and the PEERtrainer family. You guys rock!

Index